Aromatherapy for the Beauty Therapist

HAIRDRESSING AND BEAUTY INDUSTRY AUTHORITY SERIES – RELATED TITLES

HAIRDRESSING

Mahogany Hairdressing: Steps to Cutting, Colouring and Finishing Hair *Martin Gannon and Richard Thompson*

Mahogany Hairdressing: Advanced Looks *Richard Thompson and Martin Gannon*

Essensuals, Next Generation Toni & Guy: Step by Step

Professional Men's Hairdressing *Guy Kemer and Jacki Wadeson*

The Art of Dressing Long Hair *Guy Kemer and Jacki Wadeson*

Patrick Cameron: Dressing Long Hair *Patrick Cameron and Jacki Wadeson*

Patrick Cameron: Dressing Long Hair Book 2 *Patrick Cameron*

Bridal Hair *Pat Dixon and Jacki Wadeson*

Trevor Sorbie: Visions in Hair *Kris Sorbie and Jacki Wadeson*

The Total Look: The Style Guide for Hair and Make-up Professionals *Ian Mistlin*

Art of Hair Colouring *David Adams and Jacki Wadeson*

Begin Hairdressing: The Official Guide to Level 1 *Martin Green*

Hairdressing – The Foundations: The Official Guide to Level 2 *Leo Palladino* (contribution Jane Farr)

Professional Hairdressing: The Official Guide to Level 3 4e *Martin Green, Lesley Kimber and Leo Palladino*

Men's Hairdressing: Traditional and Modern Barbering 2e *Maurice Lister*

African-Caribbean Hairdressing 2e *Sandra Gittens*

Salon Management *Martin Green*

eXtensions: The Official Guide to Hair Extensions *Theresa Bullock*

BEAUTY THERAPY

Beauty Basics – The Official Guide to Level 1 *Lorraine Nordmann*

Beauty Therapy – The Foundations: The Official Guide to Level 2 *Lorraine Nordmann*

Professional Beauty Therapy: The Official Guide to Level 3 *Lorraine Nordmann, Lorraine Williamson, Pamela Linforth and Jo Crowder*

Aromatherapy for the Beauty Therapist *Valerie Ann Worwood*

Indian Head Massage *Muriel Burnham-Airey and Adele O'Keefe*

The Official Guide to Body Massage *Adele O'Keefe*

An Holistic Guide to Anatomy and Physiology *Tina Parsons*

The Encyclopedia of Nails *Jacqui Jefford and Anne Swain*

Nail Artistry *Jacqui Jefford, Sue Marsh and Anne Swain*

The Complete Nail Technician *Marian Newman*

The World of Skin Care: A Scientific Companion *Dr John Gray*

Safety in the Salon *Elaine Almond*

An Holistic Guide to Reflexology *Tina Parsons*

Nutrition: A Practical Approach *Suzanne Le Quesne*

An Holistic Guide to Massage *Tina Parsons*

The Spa Book: The Official Guide to Spa Therapy *Jane Crebbin-Bailey, Dr John Harcup and John Harrington*

Aromatherapy for the Beauty Therapist

VALERIE ANN WORWOOD

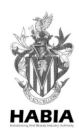

HABIA
Hairdressing And Beauty Industry Authority

THOMSON

Australia · Canada · Mexico · Singapore · Spain · United Kingdom · United States

THOMSON

Aromatherapy for the Beauty Therapist

Copyright © Valerie Ann Worwood 2001

The Thomson logo is a registered trademark used herein under licence.

For more information, contact Thomson Learning, High Holborn House, 50-51 Bedford Row, London WC1R 4LR or visit us on the World Wide Web at: http://www.thomson-learning.co.uk

British Library Cataloguing-in-Publication Data
A catalogue record for this book is available from the British Library

ISBN-13: 978-1-86152-663-2
ISBN-10: 1-86152-663-6

First edition published 2001 by Thomson Learning
Reprinted 2002 and 2005 (twice) by Thomson Learning

Typeset by Meridian Colour Repro Ltd, Pangbourne-on-Thames, Berkshire
Printed in Croatia by Zrinski d.d.

Contents

List of Illustrations

All recommendation herein contained are believed to be effective for the purposes outlined and was believed to be correct at the time of writing. Since the actual use of essential oils by others is beyond the authors and publishers control, no expressed or implied guarantee as to the effects of use can be given nor liability taken. Any recommendations set forth in the following pages is at the readers sole discretion. The author and publisher disclaim any liability arising directly or indirectly from the use of this book and assume no responsibility for any actions taken.

Preface

As a lecturer and practitioner in aromatherapy I have become acutely aware of the need for comprehensive information directly related to the growing use of essential oils within the professional beauty industry. Since the publication of my book *The Fragrant Pharmacy* in 1990, which included a chapter about the cosmetic uses of essential oils, I have received many letters from lecturers and professional beauty therapists asking me to write a book directed at the beauty therapy student and practising beauty therapist.

This book has been written specifically for the beauty therapist with the intention of providing a comprehensive and practical guide to aesthetic aromatherapy. It fills the gap between beauty therapy and aromatherapy education, and contains material never previously published. It is a source of reference on the subject of aesthetic aromatherapy for students, practising therapists, and lecturers and teachers.

Most aromatherapy texts have been written with little regard for the use of essential oils in the professional beauty salon and in aesthetic care. This book changes that, and includes only the aesthetic uses of essential oils in treatments which can be undertaken by the qualified professional, as well as specific skin-care information in the individual essential oil profiles.

Aromatherapy for the Beauty Therapist has relevance for all students studying for NVQ/SVQ Level 3, City and Guilds Certificates in Beauty Therapy, International Health and Beauty Council Diplomas, The British Association of Beauty Therapy and Cosmetology, C.I.D.E.S.C.O., BTEC National Diploma in Beauty Therapy, ITEC Diplomas in related subjects, and those studying to become aromatherapists with diplomas recognised by The International Federation of Aromatherapists, the Register of Qualified Aromatherapists, The International Society of Professional Aromatherapists and the Aromatherapy Organisations Council, as well as related overseas organisations.

Valerie Ann Worwood

Aesthetic Aromatherapy

The word 'aesthetic' means 'pertaining to the appreciation of the beautiful'. When applied to aromatherapy, 'aesthetic' means the use of essential oils, with specialist methods of application, for the purpose of improving the condition – the look and feel – of a person's face, body and hair. And, because particular aromas can enhance a person's sense of well-being, that is an integral part of aesthetic aromatherapy too.

Aesthetic aromatherapy includes facial and body treatments and cosmetics, but these are only one aspect of aromatherapy. At one time the beautifully fragranced essential oils were the main ingredient of perfumes, and they continue to be so in the more expensive perfumes produced today. Some companies have started to specialise in making entirely natural perfumes using essential oils, and this is one aspect of aromatherapy. The more commonly available form of aromatherapy today is as complementary medicine, usually involving body-work techniques.

During the early years of human development, people were impressed by the fact that certain plants produce delicious and pleasing fragrances. Religious connotations were ascribed to them, and the history of religion is also a history of fragrance. In Egyptian, Mesopotamian and Jewish cultures, fragrant plant materials were burnt as incense. Roman Catholic and Orthodox Christian churches still burn huge amounts of frankincense and myrrh during services, while Buddhist, Hindu and Shinto shrines in Asia are incomplete without a profusion of incense sticks and cones, or burning raw resin. This spiritual aspect of 'aroma-therapy' has the longest continuous tradition, dating back at least 5000 years. The Egyptians also appreciated the medicinal and preservative nature of certain fragrant plant materials. Health during life, and mummification after death, would have been impossible without them.

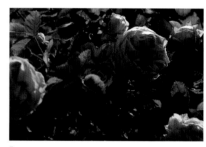

Rose

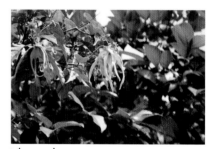

Ylang-ylang

The Egyptians also started the practice of using fragrant plant essences as perfumes, and the greatest advocate of this was Queen Cleopatra who, according to legend, had the sails of her barge soaked in rose-water, so that her intended lover, Mark Anthony – who was waiting on the shore to meet her for the first time – would smell the sweet fragrance of rose wafting on the air, prior to her arrival. Cleopatra designed a massive garden specifically built for growing fragrant plant materials, which she enthusiastically employed in her beauty and seduction methods. Cleopatra was a very intelligent woman, and is reputed to have been able to speak nine languages. Although not particularly beautiful, she made herself irresistibly attractive not only to Mark Anthony, but to the Emperor Julius Caesar himself. She wrote a *Book on Beautification*, which included recipes, although only fragments of the text now remain in existence.

As they lived in a very hot, dry environment, it was important to the ancient Egyptians that they could keep their skin supple with the use of oils. In the reign of Rameses, the monument builders even went on strike because, as they wrote, 'we have no ointments'.

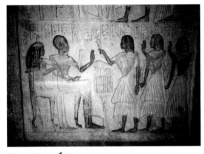

Egyptian frieze

Perfumed oils were made by steeping fragrant material in oils or fats (enfleurage); by putting the plants in hot oils and straining (maceration); or by squeezing or pressing the material (expression) using specially designed equipment. The resulting materials were stored in cool alabaster jars and used as perfumes, and face and body oils. When Tutankhamun's tomb was opened 2200 years after his death, the aroma of some of these well-stored oils could still be detected.

In 2201 B.C., a Mesopotamian book, *The Herbal of Isin*, detailed the use of 250 plants, and included recipes for perfumes and 'ointments'. The methods they used to make perfumes were recorded on brick tablets. The 7th century B.C. Assyrians loved perfumery too, and their recipes for skin and hair products still remain in existence.

There is evidence that some distillation took place in ancient Mongolian China, in the 2500 B.C. Indus Valley civilisation in Pakistan, and in the ancient Babylonian and Greek cultures. It became a much more common practice, however, after discoveries in Alexandria, Egypt, between 50 B.C. and A.D. 300. Aromatherapy took a great leap forward with distillation, because more medicinal and beautifying uses could be found for the plants processed in this way.

If we define aromatherapy as the use of distilled or otherwise processed fragrant plant material, the practice is as old as history itself. Most people in the known world aspired to acquire the precious fragrances that could improve the quality of their lives in so many different ways. The only exception to this general trend was a thousand-year period in Europe, up to the Middle Ages – which started as an early Christian Church backlash against the decadent Roman Empire's extravagant use of perfumes. During this time, the use of perfumed oils and cosmetics was kept very much alive by the Arabian cultures.

In Europe, interest in perfumed materials was rekindled in the 11th and 12th centuries by the delicious scents brought back from the East by returning Crusaders. Trade routes were opened up, and Europeans became as enthusiastic about fragrance as their Eastern neighbours. Indeed, by the 17th century no English family of any standing would be without their own personal distillation room, where perfumes and fragrant healing oils would be produced for the household's use. Modern aromatherapy is not, therefore, defined as the time when fragrance material was first used as medicine, perfume or in beauty products, but as the time when scientific investigation gave aromatherapy a new impetus – and that dates from the early 20th century.

MODERN AROMATHERAPY

The word 'aromatherapy' comes from the title of a book, *Aromathérapie*, written by a French chemist and perfumer, René-Maurice Gattefossé, and published in 1937. His story is part of aromatherapy legend, and it began in July 1910, with a accident at work:

In my personal experience, after a laboratory explosion covered me with burning substances which I extinguished by rolling on a grassy lawn, both my hands were covered with a rapidly developing gas gangrene. Just one rinse with lavender essence stopped 'the gasification of the tissue'.

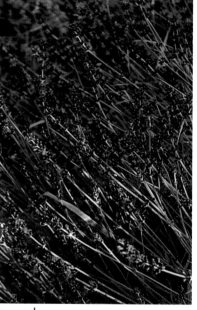

Lavender

Gattefossé was so impressed by the fact that lavender essential oil could effectively deal with this very serious condition, he started to investigate the chemical and healing properties of essential oils. He also drew on the experience of doctors using essential oils at the time, including those who had great success in healing soldiers' wounds during the First World War.

While gathering data on essential oils, Gattefossé had found they had a significant role in the field of dermatology, and after carrying out research in his own laboratory into the therapeutic action of essential oils on the skin, he published *Beauty Products* in 1936, and *Physiological Aesthetics* in 1938.

Gattefossé is often called 'the father of aromatherapy' because he was a dynamic all-rounder in the field. As a perfumer, he wrote many books about distillation and the methods of perfume manufacture, as well as playing a large part in developing essential oil cultivation and production in both France and French North Africa. He recognised the potential of essential oils in beauty, and championed percutaneous (trans-dermal) absorption as a means of applying essential oils. In all areas, he worked tirelessly to prove the beneficial effects of aromatherapy.

The continuing development of French aromatherapy, which has very much been based on clinical research and the experience of doctors, is due in large part to Gattefossé. Another classic work in the French medical tradition was *The Practice of Aromatherapy* by Dr Jean Valnet, first published in 1980.

Aromatherapy is a developing art and science. As time goes on and further scientific research and empirical experience are acquired, it becomes increasingly clear that, in essential oils, nature blessed humanity with a set of exquisite tools to greatly improve our well-being – in the field of beauty, as in other ways.

BEAUTY AND AESTHETIC TREATMENTS

In 1550 B.C. there appeared in ancient Egypt a document entitled *Eber's Papyrus*. As well as containing many health remedies, it listed 22 cosmetics. A slightly later document, the *Smith Surgical Papyrus*, contained a section called 'Transforming an Old Man into a Youth'. In all the ancient cultures there were people who wrote at length about the beautifying properties of fragrant materials. In ancient Rome, for example, Kriton – the Empress Plotina's physician – wrote several books on cosmetics, which included recipes for wrinkle and freckle removers, face-waters, pomades, perfumed oils, hair removers, and perfumes for the body, bed and clothing.

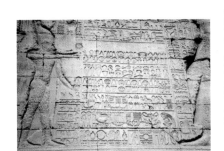

Temple at Edfu, Egypt – depicting fragrance recipes

Clearly, throughout time, people have sought to be more beautiful and youthful-looking, and they often used aromatics and essential oils. In the 1856 edition of *The Art of Perfumery*, for example, Septimus Piesse* gave this recipe for Rose Cold Cream, using rose otto:

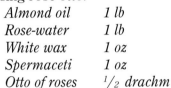

Almond oil	*1 lb*
Rose-water	*1 lb*
White wax	*1 oz*
Spermaceti	*1 oz*
Otto of roses	*$^1/_2$ drachm*

Spermaceti is a soft, white fatty substance that comes from the head of the sperm-whale. It needs to be refined before use. It was once widely used in medicinal preparations and candle-making.

During the 19th and early 20th century natural ingredients, whether from plants or animals, were replaced by the ingenious inventions of a new profession – cosmetic chemists. Products with natural ingredients came to be seen as less 'modern', and were replaced with ingredients with impressive-sounding scientific names.

These mass-marketed products became the norm, while beauty therapy treatments using pure essential oils became ever more rare, and very much the exclusive privilege of the wealthy. By the 1970s few people still appreciated the remarkable capacity of essential oils to beautify the skin and bring a lustrous glow to the body, and those who did could command high prices for their treatments. One of these pioneers was Marguerite Maury, a French woman who had salons in Switzerland and, eventually, London. With a specialisation in rejuvenation and revitalisation, she combined beauty therapy techniques with essential oils, and popularised – amongst those 'in the know' – body massage using essential oils.

Maury was initially invited to London to lecture and hold workshops for interested beauty therapists and in 1960 her book,

---

*Septimus Piesse, *The Art of Perfumery*, London: Longman Brown Green Longmans & Roberts, 1856 (2nd edition).

The Secret of Life and Youth, was translated from French into English. This was the start of aromatherapy for a larger audience in Britain. Micheline Arcier worked alongside Maury, and later opened her own aromatherapy salon. Danielle Ryman, as a young woman, became Maury's assistant in London, and carried on Maury's work after her death. London soon developed a reputation among the European rich and famous as the place to go to for aesthetic aromatherapy treatments.

Today, aromatherapy is used in beauty and aesthetic treatments for relaxation, stress-relief, rejuvenation and revitalisation, uplifting massage treatment, specific beauty and skin condition treatments including facials, and in slimming treatments. Essential oils are found as ingredients in all manner of beauty products, including face creams and lotions, face scrubs, masks, and toners, body lotions of all kinds, slimming treatments, sun tanning and protection products, and pedicure and manicure products.

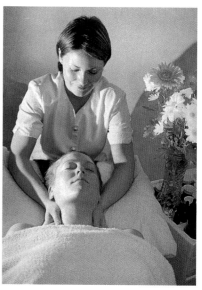

Aromatherapy treatment salon

HAIRDRESSING

Modern aromatherapy treatments are an expansion of the age-old practice of adding natural plant ingredients to washing and hairdressing procedures. Most people know that camomile flowers or lemon will lighten blonde hair, and that a rosemary rinse will keep oily hair in good condition, and make it shine. For this reason, rosemary water has been prepared by women in kitchens all over the world for centuries. In 1856, they were recommended by Piesse to use 10 lb of rosemary 'free from stalk' in 12 gallons of water, and to 'draw off by distillation ten gallons'.

Today, the shelves are packed with products claiming to include among their ingredients natural plant materials. Indeed, it is hard to find a hair product that doesn't boast some plant material is contained within it. However, a quick educated look at the ingredients will soon tell you that the plant addition is in such small quantities that it will do little for the hair, although it no doubt does a great deal for the marketing. When a product claims to be 'aromatherapy' and, for example, 'stimulating' or 'relaxing', it often contains the essential oils in such minute quantities that the aroma is undetectable and a synthetic fragrance is added for effect. Worse is when the ingredient is no more than a synthetic chemical copying the fragrance of an essential oil, and has none of its therapeutic qualities.

However, there are a few genuine aromatherapy products on the market, not only for washing and conditioning the hair, but to encourage hair regrowth, as well as those designed as scalp tonics and to be helpful in certain scalp conditions.

FRAGRANCES

The word 'perfume' comes from the Latin *per fumin*, which means 'by smoke', because burning fragrant plant material was the first way in which people discovered that the aroma in certain plants could be released by heat. All the early civilisations loved

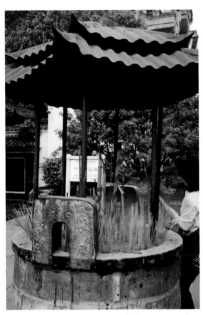
Burning incense at Buddhist temple

perfumes, which were a very precious commodity at the time. In 300 B.C. the ancient Greek, Theophrastus, wrote a book called *Concerning Odours*, which not only gave instructions on how to make perfumes, but listed their medicinal and other properties. He wondered 'why is it that perfumes appear to be sweetest when the scent comes from the wrist?'

During the last years of the ancient Egyptian era, there was a fusion of Egyptian and Greek culture, and a wide range of perfumes became available. Writers of the time name around 30 perfumes, some of which were used as cosmetics, others for sprinkling on bed-linen or clothes, while others were designed for medicinal use.

We know from written records that the perfume material available to the ancient Greeks included cassia, cinnamon, cardamom, carnation, spikenard, storax, iris, saffron, myrrh, ginger-grass, sweet flag, sweet marjoram, lotus, dill, rose, lilies, myrtle, bergamot, bay, mint, thyme, hyacinth, violets and narcissus. These were made into essences, or incorporated into oils and unguents using olive, sesame, castor and linseed oils. Wine was another popular 'carrier' of fragrant material.

COMPLEMENTARY MEDICINE

Aromatherapy has become such a popular form of complementary medicine because, correctly used, it provides a safe and effective method of improving health. The hundred or so essential oils in common use provide, between them, the means of approaching many diverse health problems. As a complementary medicine, aromatherapy employs many more essential oils than would be used in beauty therapy. In general, beauty therapists would only use oils which are effective in skin care and other beauty-related treatments, and would not be concerned with the wider range of medical therapeutic properties available from different essential oils. The glossary below lists physical effects required from aromatherapy practised as a complementary medicine, and is included only as a reference for the wider effects available from the use of essential oils. Clearly, you would not expect one essential oil to be able to perform all the physical effects listed below. An essential oil may have one or more of these properties.

Glossary of Therapeutic Properties

Medical Terminology	Physical Effect
Analgesic	reduces pain sensation
Antibiotic/anti-bacterial	prevents bacterial growth
Anti-fungal	prevents fungal growth
Anti-infectious	prevents uptake of infection
Anti-parasitic	acts against insect parasites
Anti-putrescent	acts against putrefaction
Antisclerotic	prevents hardening of cells and tissues
Antiseptic	destroys microbes and prevents their development
Anti-spasmodic	prevents or relieves spasms, convulsions or contractions
Anti-sudorific	prevents sweating
Antitussive	relieves coughs
Anti-viral	prevents viral growth
Balsamic	soothing to sore throats, coughs etc.
Calmative	sedative, calming agent
Carminative	relieves flatulence, easing abdominal pain and bloating
Cholagogue	promotes the evacuation of bile from gall bladder and ducts
Cicatrisive	promotes the formation of scar tissue, thus healing
Cytophylactic	promotes cell turnover, thus healing
Depurative	cleanser, detoxifier; purifies blood and internal organs
Diuretic	promotes the removal of excess water from the body by urine
Emmenagogue	induces or regularises menstruation
Emollient	soothes and softens skin
Expectorant	promotes removal of mucus from the body
Febrifuge	an anti-febrile (anti-fever) agent
Galactagogue	induces the flow of milk
Haemostatic	stops bleeding
Hepatic	acts on the liver
Immuno-stimulant	stimulates the action of the immune system
Mucolytic	breaks down mucous
Nervine	acts on nerves; relieves nervous disorders
Pectoral	beneficial for diseases or conditions of the chest and respiratory system
Rubefacient	a counter-irritant producing redness of the skin
Sedative	reduces mental excitement or physical ctivity
Soporific	induces, or tends to induce sleep
Stimulant	increases overall function of the body
Stomachic	good for the stomach; gastric tonic, digestive aid
Tonic	invigorates, refreshes and restores body functions
Vermifuge	expels intestinal worms
Vulnerary	heals wounds and sores by external application

CONTEMPORARY PSYCHOLOGY

Aroma psychology specifically refers to the use of essential oils to positively affect the mind – such as memory enhancement, learning improvement, mood uplifting and confidence boosting. These mental stimulations have a direct impact on daily performance and practical applications are currently being used by a wide range of organisations.

A new branch of psychology called *Aroma-Genera* utilises the ability of certain blends of essential oil to access deeply held memories. It releases the emotions that are attached to experiences of past events. The wider use of aroma in psychology of the future can be anticipated.

How Aromatherapy Works

There are three ways in which essential oil molecules enter the body and have an effect on it: by inhalation, by trans-dermal absorption and for medical practitioner by ingestion. In a general sense, aromatherapy increases blood supply to the tissues, which helps the proliferation of cells and regeneration, increasing oxygenation and lymphatic flow. Aromatherapy thus leads to an internal and external revitalisation and radiance, improving self-confidence – the ultimate aid to beauty. In addition, specific essential oils can also have a direct effect on particular skin conditions.

Because the skin is on the surface of the body, and easily seen, the effect that essential oils have on it is easily observable; but once inside the body, essential oils also have an effect on the hormones, nerves, tissues and organs, as well as on the mind and emotions. Aromatherapy is called a holistic therapy because it can affect a person in many different ways, all at the same time.

INHALATION

When we inhale essential oils, they are absorbed by the delicate membranes of the nose, bronchioles (air tubes) and lungs. In this way they can enter the bloodstream. Many drugs are now administered by inhalation, including those for asthma, emphysema, bronchitis and anaesthesia.

THE SENSE OF SMELL

Essential oils have an effect on the emotions most obviously because the smell mechanism, the olfactory organs, are actually part of the brain, and aroma sets off an immediate reaction in the brain. For example, if a stranger passes you on the street wearing the same perfume or eau de cologne regularly worn by a person you know, you'll subconsciously be reminded of that person, and instantly think about them.

When we smell a familiar aroma, the emotions associated with it return too. If the person we associate with a particular fragrance was a loving friend, positive emotions will return with their memory. If, on the other hand, the person was physically or emotionally violent towards us, the fragrance could trigger a reoccurrence of the negative emotions we felt in that person's presence.

Each individual person has an aroma-history that a therapist cannot be aware of. Even the client themselves may not realise that a particular aroma reminds them of a negative incident or person in their past. For this reason, if a client says they really don't like a particular aroma, that must be respected and an alternative essential oil found.

It has been estimated that the human nose is capable of distinguishing between 10000 different smells. The exact physiological mechanism of smell is still a scientific mystery, although certain facts are known:

- We inhale aromatic molecules that are floating in the air. A flower is only fragrant if it releases aromatic molecules into the atmosphere around it.
- These molecules float into the nasal cavity and come into contact with two small areas at the top, packed with tufts of cilia embedded in watery mucous. The cilia are attached to 'stalks' (called *dendrites* or *olfactory nerve processes*) which pass through the thin bony plate (*cribiform plate* of the *ethmoid* bone) at the top of the nasal cavity.
- When an aromatic molecule touches the cilia, chemical and electrical activity is triggered, causing a message to be sent to the brain. The message starts with the cilia (or *olfactory receptors*), and then travels along the dendrites, via mitral cells, to the olfactory bulb – and the brain.

The most remarkable thing about the olfactory system is that it is actually a part of the brain. When we talk about the sense of smell, we are discussing brain cells. Although the brain is usually thought of as a distinct mass, there is an extension to it, right at the top of the nose – the olfactory bulb. This protrudes from the brain, looking rather like two tiny upside-down spoons. It is from this extraordinary organ that the dendrites extend downward, through the thin bony plate, ending in the cilia inside the top of the nasal cavity.

Brain cells in general do not replace themselves if damaged, but the olfactory cells do. This is an important survival mechanism because the cilia are relatively exposed, and vulnerable to attack by all manner of dangerous microbes and toxic gases. If they did not regenerate themselves, we might all lose our sense of smell after coming into contact with air-borne viruses, or being too long in a polluted or toxic atmosphere. And the sense of smell is really vital to survival as it tells us that food is available, or that we are in danger – from fire for example. However, despite the fact that olfactory cells are capable of regenerating themselves, many people have completely lost their sense of smell, often for unknown reasons. These people are known as *anosmic*, and more often than not, there is little that modern medicine can do to remedy their situation. Anosmia not only denies these people the

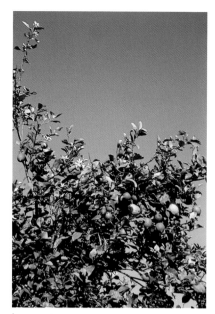
Lemon tree

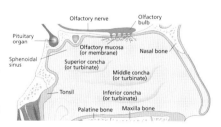
Nose/olfaction

ACTIVITY

Close your eyes, and imagine biting into one half of a fresh, juicy lemon. Inhale the fresh aroma.

Notice what physiological change is happening within your mouth. Has it produced more saliva than usual?

(The thought of the smell of the lemon is sufficient to activate the mind–body connection, and more saliva than normal is produced.)

pleasures associated with smell and taste, but can also lead to depression and depressive disorders.

THE SKIN AND ITS STRUCTURE

The skin is the largest organ of the human body, and performs many functions:

- it cushions the body against external forces;
- it provides waterproof protection through the lubricating activity of the sebaceous glands that produce sebum;
- it helps retain vital fluids within the body;
- it regulates temperature – cooling the body when it is hot and conserving heat when it is cold: when hot, the sweat glands produce perspiration, and the blood vessels widen (dilate) to dissipate heat; when cold, the blood vessels narrow (constrict) to conserve body heat;
- it shields internal organs from harmful rays from the sun;
- it provides a barrier against bacteria, viruses, other micro-organisms and chemical pollutants;
- it contains many cells that identify – touch, pain, pressure, itching;
- it excretes waste and toxins.

Structure of the Skin

The skin has several layers and sits on muscle which is covered by subcutaneous fat. In this fat layer there are blood vessels, and the roots of the hair follicles and sweat glands.

Epidermis

The epidermis is the tough outer layer of skin. It is much thinner than the dermis. Passing through the epidermis are hair follicles and sweat glands – which form the pores at the skin surface. The cells of the epidermis are in a constant process of change, taking around 28 days to progress from the inner, more active level, to the outer, dead, surface. The living cells at the innermost level produce a hard protein, keratin, which toughens the epidermis. These cells divide very rapidly at this stage, eventually slowing down and forming a transitional level between the inner and outer epidermis. Finally, these transitional cells die, and are pushed towards the surface by active cells below. All skin cells at the body surface are dead, and are constantly shed. Ninety per cent of household dust is said to be dead skin cells.

Active (Basal) Cell Layer

This very thin layer separates the outer epidermis from the inner dermis. The nerves of touch sensation stop at this layer, not passing through it. This layer contains desquamating cells which regulate the skin-shedding process. In black skins, desquamating cells contain pigmentary cells called melanocytes, which produce melanin and give colour to the epidermal cells.

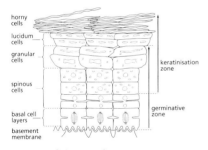

horny cells
lucidum cells
granular cells
keratinisation zone
spinous cells
germinative zone
basal cell layers
basement membrane

Layers of the epidermis

Dermis

The dermis is the inner, thicker layer of living skin. It is made of connective tissue, interspersed with specialist nerves and other cells. Passing through the dermis are blood capillaries, hair follicles, sebaceous glands, sweat glands and nerves. It also contains hair erector muscle, and specialist nerves to detect heat, cold and various kinds of touch sensation.

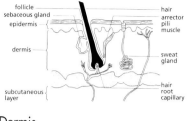

Dermis

Trans-Dermal Absorption

The fact that substances can be passed through the skin and into the underlying blood vessels is utilised by drug manufacturers who produce trans-dermal patches, or 'skin patches' – adhesive, drug-impregnated pads which are attached to the skin. Nicotine patches are perhaps the best known example of this relatively new drug-delivery system, but there are many others, including those for angina, terminal pain, travel sickness and hormone replacement therapy.

Essential oils are thought to enter the skin in several ways. They may enter through hair follicles or sweat glands, and gain access to blood vessels through the capillary network. When diluted in a vegetable oil or other carrier and applied to the skin, only the extremely small essential oil molecules pass into the skin. It is thought they pass so efficiently through tissue because they can penetrate the fatty layers and travel through the interstitial fluid (which surrounds all body cells). Some essential oils with smaller molecules may also travel transcellularly, that is, directly through the cell.

The ability of essential oils to travel through body tissue is well documented, and it has been shown that essential oil components applied through massage can be detected in body waste such as urine, faeces and perspiration, and in the outward breath. This permeating ability of essential oils has stimulated medical researchers to explore the possibility of using essential oils as vehicles on which to attach pharmaceutical drugs, which can 'piggy back' on the essential oils and be carried inside the body.

> **ACTIVITY**
> Put a dab of lavender essential oil on your outer cheek and wait a few minutes. You will soon taste the lavender inside your mouth. This is not only because you can smell the lavender, but because the essential oil has actually passed through the tissue.

THE CIRCULATORY/CARDIOVASCULAR SYSTEM

The heart pumps blood through a system of vessels, providing the skin and other tissues with oxygen, nutrients and hormones, and carrying away waste products, which are excreted by the kidneys. Good blood circulation is vital to health as it affects the working of every organ of the body, including the brain.

Some essential oils stimulate blood circulation, allowing a more efficient disposal of unwanted matter, including carbon dioxide and other waste products of cell metabolism. The immune system is improved by the general increase in blood movement, and blood viscosity is decreased.

Suggested oils are: geranium, rose, cypress and vetiver.

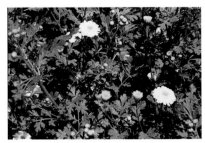

Lymph vessels

Diagram labels:
- right lymphatic duct
- right subclavian vein
- submandibular lymph node
- deep cervical lymph nodes
- internal jugular vein
- left subclavian vein
- axillary lymph node
- thoracic duct
- intestinal lymph nodes
- inguinal lymph nodes
- iliac nodes

THE LYMPHATIC SYSTEM

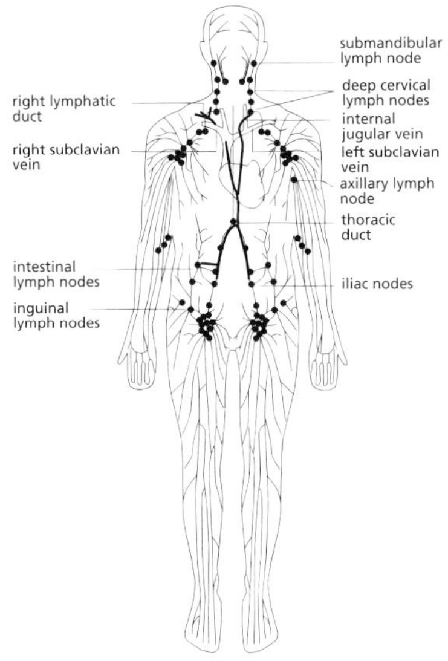

Lymph is a colourless body fluid that contains fats, proteins and white blood cells called lymphocytes. It is constantly transported throughout the body by a system of vessels called lymphatics. The lymphatic system has no central pumping machine (as the heart provides for blood circulation). There are one-way valves in the lymphatics, ensuring the lymphatic fluid only moves in one direction, and motion is caused by the regular movement of the body's muscles.

The lymphatic system is part of the body's immune system. It includes lymph nodes, which are nodules packed with white blood cells that destroy bacteria, viruses and various other micro-organisms, as well as other harmful matter. All body tissues have a certain amount of lymphatic fluid around them – providing oxygen and nutrients, as well as a 'clean-up' service. Lymphatic fluid is derived from the bloodstream, to which it eventually returns. Indeed, during the course of a single day around 24 litres (5.28 gallons) of lymphatic fluid will pass from the bloodstream, via the walls of capillaries, to body tissues; while 20 litres (4.40 gallons) of lymph will return to the bloodstream via the same route, and 4 litres (0.88 gallons) will return to the lymphatic system.

Suggested oils are: thyme linalol, niaouli, lemon and frankincense.

THE NERVOUS SYSTEM

The nervous system is in two parts: the central nervous system (CNS) and the peripheral nervous system (PNS). The CNS consists of the brain, and the brainstem which runs through the vertebrae. The CNS contains the nerve cells that receive information, analyse it and send out an appropriate response. The PNS radiates outward from the brainstem to every part of the body, and carries the messages to and from the CNS.

The peripheral nervous system has three parts, all of which are directly affected by the action of essential oils. One branch of the PNS is in the head and includes – as well as the nerves activating the eyes, ears and taste buds – the nose and olfactory system. Essential oils initiate electro-chemical messages being sent to the limbic portion of the brain, stimulating memory, mood and emotion.

Another part of the PNS extends to the skin and muscles. Essential oils are well known to have a direct impact on the ability of muscles to relax, which is a feature of the nervous system. Some essential oil components have a remarkable ability to penetrate all layers of the skin.

The third branch of the PNS is the autonomic or involuntary nervous system, itself consisting of two parts: the sympathetic and parasympathetic, which work like a pair of on–off switches, keeping certain parts of the body working in balance. In the 1980s Professor Torii of Toho University in Japan showed that certain

Camomile roman

essential oils increased the action of the sympathetic nervous system, while others decreased it. On all fronts then, essential oils can be seen to have a direct effect on the nervous system.

Suggested oils are: bergamot, camomile roman, lavender and sandalwood.

THE ENDOCRINE SYSTEM

Normal body functioning is to a very large degree regulated by hormones. Many hormones are produced by the endocrine system of glands, including the pituitary, thyroid, parathyroid, adrenal cortex, ovaries, testes and pancreas. Hormones are also produced by nerve impulse transmission, and even the heart produces its own hormones.

Certain essential oils are known as 'phyto-hormones', indicating these plant substances (*phyto-*) can mimic in some respects the activity of human hormones.

The skin is affected by hormonal activity. Some women find their skin condition changing at different times of the menstrual cycle, or during menopause; while the onset of adolescence, which is a time of exceptional hormonal activity, can cause spots or acne. Using certain essential oils in beauty therapy can act as a harmoniser of hormones, leading to an improvement of the skin condition.

Suggested oils are: clary sage, fennel, geranium and ylang-ylang.

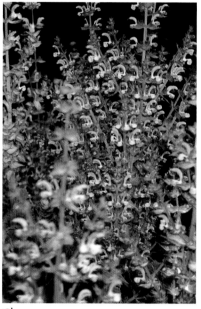

Clary sage

THE MUSCULAR SYSTEM

Muscles are collections of specialised cells capable of contraction and relaxation. There are 600 *skeletal* muscles in the human body, as well as the *smooth* muscles of internal organs, and the *cardiac* muscle of the heart.

Beauty therapy is concerned with the action of the skeletal muscles, which cover the body, and lie under the skin in the face and neck. Small muscles consist of just a few bundles of fibres, while larger muscles consist of hundreds of bundles. Each muscle fibre is made up of myofibrils, arranged in a longitudinal pattern, and these are composed of two types of protein filament, actin and myosin, which control the action of contraction.

Essential oils serve to relax and release tension in constricted muscles, giving tone and firm appearance to muscles in the face. Both massage and essential oils help to decongest muscles, releasing lactic acid and uric acid held in them.

Suggested oils are: rosemary, marjoram, black pepper and ginger.

THE DIGESTIVE SYSTEM

The digestive system is concerned with the processing of food and drink. It is composed of the oesophagus, stomach, duodenum, small intestine and colon. Certain essential oils have the effect of relaxing muscles concerned with the digestive system, and releasing trapped wind. Other essential oils are diuretic, and help the elimination of fluids from the body, through the urinary system.

Suggested oils are: coriander, dill, juniper and peppermint.

THE RESPIRATORY SYSTEM

Respiration is the means by which oxygen is supplied to body cells, and carbon dioxide is expelled. Air is inhaled through the nose and mouth, travels down the trachea to the bronchus, the smaller bronchiole, and to the lungs. The working mechanism of the lung is made up of millions of tiny balloon-like sacs called alveoli. These are arranged in groups, and are extremely well supplied with a complex network of capillaries, linking the alveoli to veins.

The role of the alveoli is to transfer oxygen from air into the bloodsteam, and to receive waste carbon dioxide from the blood, so it can be expelled. They do this by a process known as diffusion, where the oxygen and carbon dioxide pass effortlessly through the thin membranous alveoli walls, the epithelium, which are composed of just one layer of cells.

When essential oils are inhaled they arrive at the alveoli then pass into the bloodstream. There is moisture present at the internal alveoli walls, which dissolves some particles before they pass through the epithelial wall. The ease with which a particular essential oil can enter the bloodstream through this route is dependent on the size and nature of its molecules.

Essential oils, being volatile, have access to the entire respiratory system, and may even enter the bloodstream through it. Within the various tubes and alveoli, the antibacterial and anti-viral qualities of essential oils can take effect, and help fight infection. Certain essential oils are also antispasmodic, and help prevent spasm in the tubes; or are expectorant, and can help release phlegm.

Suggested oils are: ravensara, eucalyptus, tea tree and myrtle.

THE REPRODUCTIVE SYSTEM

The reproductive system involves those organs related to sexuality and reproduction. In women, this includes the ovaries, fallopian tubes, uterus and vagina; and in men, the seminal vesicles, vas deferens, prostate gland, testes and penis.

Each 28-day cycle, or thereabouts, the lining of the uterus, the endometrium, is shed. The reproductive cycle can cause difficulties such as dysmenorrhoea, menorrhagia, amenorrhoea, back ache, constipation or diarrhoea, stress and skin problems. Essential oils have long been used to treat women for these difficulties, as well as during pregnancy and labour.

Suggested oils are: rose, geranium, camomile roman and fennel.

THE SKELETAL SYSTEM

The skeletal system consists of 213 bones, containing mostly calcium and phosphorus. Inside the central cavity of some bones, and in the spaces of the inner layer of spongy bone, is a fatty tissue called bone marrow, in which red blood cells, platelets and most white cells are formed.

Certain essential oils used to help in the healing process of broken bones are thought to be effective because of their electrical activity. Inflammation of the joints is successfully treated with anti-inflammatory essential oils.

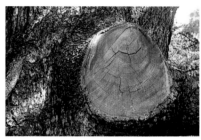
Cedarwood (wood)

Suggested oils are (bones): ginger, black pepper, cedarwood and yarrow.
Suggested oils are (anti-inflammatory): yarrow, camomile german and camomile roman.

CHAPTER 2

Safety and Contra-Indications

Essential oils are effective because they are highly active plant substances, with the ability to cause physiological changes within the human body. The three rules of safe essential oils are:

- *purity of product* – use only pure, therapeutic-quality essential oils;
- *informed use* – ascertain the correct essential oil for the condition or treatment;
- *correct dose* – use the correct dosages for the condition or treatment.

The use of essential oils in aesthetic aromatherapy will differ from that used in clinical aromatherapy or aromatic medicine. Clinical aromatherapists use essential oils, administrative methods and dosage levels that are unsuitable for use in aesthetic aromatherapy. The beauty therapist should not attempt to treat any medical conditions unless she is also a professionally qualified aromatherapist, registered with a recognised professional body.

For their personal safety, the therapist should:

- wash all traces of essential oil from the hands before touching eyes or face;
- ensure the working area is well ventilated;
- drink at least half a litre of water during the working day;
- take the time to inhale fresh air as often as possible through the working day.

AREAS OF CAUTION

Essential oils are scientifically tested in their undiluted form to determine their potential harmful effects. Increasing amounts of essential oil are applied to the skin, or given orally, to determine how much can be administered. In aesthetic aromatherapy, where just a few drops from one bottle are likely to be used on the skin in a diluted form, the actual potential for harm is low. This is not to say that caution should not always be employed.

FIRST AID
- If essential oils get in the **eyes**: rinse thoroughly with water.
- If **skin irritation** occurs, apply large amounts of plain vegetable oil.
- If blending, ensure there is adequate **ventilation**.

Dermal Tests

Essential oils are widely used by the perfumery and cosmetic industries, who must consider that a customer might be using one of their products every day, over perhaps many years. Aesthetic therapists are concerned with the irritant and sensitisation potential of essential oils, as they apply them to the skin. The tests measure:

- **irritation** – localised sensitivity at site of application;
- **sensitisation** – allergic reaction involving immune system;
- **photosensitivity** – localised sensitivity due to ultra-violet rays, including those from the sun.

Irritation

This is a local reaction of the skin to a substance. It may manifest as itching, a rash, a burning sensation, inflammation or soreness. It affects the area of the skin on which the essential oil was applied; it does not affect other parts of the body.

- Certain essential oils are known to have skin irritation effects, and should be avoided or used with caution. These are: *clove (all types), cinnamon bark, cinnamon leaf and oregano.*
- The following essential oils should be used with care, especially on persons with sensitive skin: *basil, rosemary, peppermint, lemongrass, verbena, fennel, sage, red thyme, aniseed, pine, pimento berry, fir and bay.*

Sensitisation

People develop allergies to all sorts of substances, including essential oils. This is known as sensitisation, which is individual-specific. A reaction may not occur on the first application of the antigen-substance, but on subsequent applications as the immune system activates the response. The allergic person may experience a mild reaction such as itching or sneezing, develop a temperature, or may react more severely, with swelling and breathing difficulties.

Clearly, making thorough notes of all known allergies at the time of the initial client consultation is important in avoiding essential oils that may have an adverse affect on a particular client. Equally important is to keep accurate client records so that if sensitisation occurs, the allergen can be identified. If a person is sensitive to one of the *resins or gums*, it is possible they will have the same reaction to all essential oils from these sources. All *cinnamon* essential oils are contra-indicated for persons with allergic tendencies. *Bay laurel* is said to create a sensitising effect when used over a period of time.

- A skin test should be carried out on people with sensitive skin or allergic reactions to aromatic materials. To conduct a skin test, put one drop of the undiluted essential oil on the fabric portion of a plaster, attach it to the inner arm of the elbow,

---

ACTIVITY

To experience the sensation of skin irritation, put a smear of neat peppermint essential oil on the back of your neck, by the hair line. Wait for a few minutes.

You may feel the skin first go cold, then begin to feel irritated and a prickling sensation.

This activity, at this amount, is not damaging to the skin.

FIRE – EMERGENCY!

To extinguish a fire involving essential oils:

- **Use** fire-fighting equipment based on carbon dioxide, dry powder, foam or vaporising liquid.
- **Do not use water**.
- Try to avoid inhaling smoke or other fumes.

ESSENTIAL OILS TO BE AVOIDED BY THOSE WITH EPILEPSY

Aniseed	Fennel	Lavendin
Basil	Hyssop	Rosemary

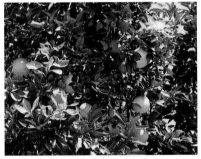

Grapefruit

and remove after 24 hours. As the skin does not always react with the first application of an allergen, a further test may be required. This can also be carried out with diluted essential oil blends.

Photosensitivity

Certain essential oils can cause a photo-chemical reaction on the skin if it is exposed to direct and intense ultra-violet (UV) rays – from the sun or tanning equipment. Bergamot and lime are more highly photosensitive than other essential oils in this group.

The result of combining the use of a photosensitive essential oil with UV exposure is usually a change of skin colour. This may be slight, or the affected area of skin may appear tanned, or there may be hyper-pigmentation. In some cases, where high quantities of undiluted essential oils are applied, skin damage such as blistering may occur. No essential oil treatments should be given before sunbed or other tanning equipment is used.

All citrus essential oils can have a degree of photosensitivity, unless especially manipulated not to do so by the removal of a group of aromatic chemicals, the furocoumarins. Such essential oils are labelled FCF, meaning furocoumarin free.

The following should not be used when going in prolonged sunlight:

- *bergamot, lime, grapefruit, orange, lemon, angelica seed, mandarin, tangerine, verbena, caraway seed, cumin seed and tagetes.*

Oral Ingestion (by Mouth) Tests

Oral testing is carried out because essential oils are used extensively by the food and drink industries. However, oral ingestion of essential oils is not within the scope of beauty therapy, and aesthetic therapists should never suggest to their clients that they take essential oils in this way. Taking essential oils orally is the most hazardous method of using essential oils.

Oral administration of essential oils is prescribed by some qualified medical aromatherapists, but this method is not generally used in aromatherapy.

ESSENTIAL OILS AND ELECTRICAL EQUIPMENT

Using essential oils may increase the physiological effects of any facial treatment equipment used, as a result of the electro-chemical nature of the aromatic compounds in essential oils. If you will be using essential oils with any electrical equipment for any form of body treatments, or in saunas and steam rooms, check with the manufacturers of the electrical equipment beforehand.

CHAPTER 3

Fixed Vegetable Oils

Essential oils must be diluted before they are used on the face or body. The medium most suitable is vegetable oil. Other mediums are pre-prepared lotions, creams and gels. Essential oils should not be used with animal fats, fish oils, mineral oils such as petroleum oil (such as 'baby oil'), or any synthetic or chemically treated vegetable oil.

VEGETABLE OILS

- Vegetable oils are obtained from:
  - either tree crops (such as almonds, hazelnuts, olives, coconut or peach kernel);
  - or oilseed crops (such as sunflowers, rapeseed or soya).
- Vegetable oils are 'fixed oils'. They do not evaporate, even when warm, and will leave a permanent oily mark if dropped on paper. Essential oils evaporate in both warm and cold conditions, and if coloured may leave a pigmentation mark. However, the majority do not leave an oily mark when dry.
- Essential oils are easily dispersed in all vegetable oils.

'CARRIER OIL' OR 'BASE OIL'?

A distinction can be drawn between vegetable oils used as a general *carrier*, and those used as a *base*.

- *Carrier oils* are those whose primary role is simply to carry the therapeutic essential oil molecules to where they are needed. The tiny amount of essential oil required in a treatment would be impossible to distribute over a large area of skin unless it was first diluted in a much larger volume of carrier oil.
- *Base oils* are individual or blends of carrier oils, which are chosen for their particular therapeutic actions. They are known to have therapeutic effects on the skin in their own right. Base oils act in synergy with essential oils to create a more effective compound. This happens in two ways:
  - base oils enhance the effect of the essential oil;
  - essential oils enhance the effect of the base oil.

In beauty therapy the subject of base oils is very important as certain pure vegetable oils have such a beneficial action on the skin. By comparison, medical/clinical aromatherapy generally

TIP

Wheatgerm oil can be used as a preservative because of its vitamin E content. Some therapists use it as 5–10 per cent of the total carrier/base oil solely for that reason.

uses vegetable carrier oils, simply as a way to deliver the essential oils.

THE IMPORTANCE OF USING PURE, ORGANIC, NATURAL VEGETABLE OILS

- *'Pure'* indicates that the oil has not been mixed with any other oil species, not been adulterated with any chemical additions, and not been through processes which would leach from it the vitamins, minerals and other positive elements that exist in natural vegetable oils.
- *Organic oils* are those extracted from plants which have not been grown with the use of pesticides, herbicides and fungicides (known collectively as *biocides*), chemical fertilisers or growth enhancers. Also, organically cultivated vegetable oils should not be genetically modified (GM).
- *Natural oils* are those which contain 100 per cent of a natural substance. Many cosmetic oils and other products contain ingredients that are *synthetic*, which means they have been man-made by scientists and chemists to certain commercial specifications.

How Pure, Organic, Natural Vegetable Oils Differ from Processed Oils

Most vegetable oils produced for the general food market are subjected to many chemical and other processes, designed to provide a colourless, odourless oil, with a long shelf-life. The processes used to obtain this product diminish the natural nutrients and health-giving properties in the oil. To distinguish these oils from 'natural' oils, they are here called 'processed' oils.

Such oils are put through a lengthy series of procedures involving the use of chemical solvents and clay-based earths to remove: *waxes, gums, lecithin, free fatty acids, monoacylglycerols, diacylglycerols, coloured compounds, odours (volatile compounds), pesticides etc.* The solvents and earths themselves have to be removed by further procedures.

Chemical Washing due to Long Storage

Many commercial vegetable oils are extracted from seeds or beans which were harvested up to two years previously, and have been in storage since that time. Fungi and mould can develop on the plant material, and this is washed off by using chemicals. Also during long storage, plant material loses its 'vibrancy' – some of its vitamins and minerals etc.

Any one 'processed' oil could have been subjected to any, or all, of the following, perhaps several times over:

Solvent Extraction

To break open the seeds and their endosperm cells (store of energy), and release the vegetable oil contained in them, the material is heated to about 100°C. It is then pressed through a filter. Some oil is extracted in this way, but a solid cake is also produced, and further processes are required to extract the oil from this.

The first process is solvent extraction. The solvent separates the oil from the solids, and the solvent–oil mix is distilled, to separate the two. The oil at this stage is known as 'crude oil' and is further processed.

Degumming (or Filtration)

The 'crude oil' is mixed with water and heated to about 80°C. It is then centrifuged, and the water-soluble elements (including lecithin) are run off.

Neutralisation

Sodium hydroxide (or sodium carbonate) solution in water is often used to convert free fatty acids into their sodium salts.

Bleaching

Clay-based earths could be used to absorb coloured material. Then the mixture is filtered to remove the earths (such as 'fullers' earth').

Deodorisation

This is the last stage of the 'refining' process. It aims to remove traces of pesticide which are volatile, along with the elements that give the oil its taste and smell. The oil is heated to 180–240°C, and put in a vacuum. Jets of highly heated steam are passed into this, and by steam distillation only those elements that have a lower boiling point than the oil itself are taken out.

Summary

- The industrial production of vegetable oils is partly determined by: the cultivation methods (the extraction of pesticides, herbicides, fungicides, chemical fertilisers and growth enhancers), partly by the commercial need for a product with a long shelf-life, and partly by the perceived customer requirement for a product that is colourless and odourless.
- The industrial production of vegetable oils involves subjecting the oil material to many chemical and heat processes.
- By comparison, pure, organic oils are produced with different customer needs. They do not need:
  – to be subjected to processes to extract chemicals used in the cultivation of the plant material;
  – to be colourless or odourless;
  – to have such a long shelf-life.
- Consequently, 'pure', 'organic' oils retain within them more of the vital nutrients of the plant material.

HEALTH AND SAFETY
Skin irritation and sensitivity may be caused by using 'processed' oils which still have residues of biocides or chemical solvents used in the oil production.

TIP
Look for vegetable oils that have one or more of the following words on their labels:
organic
unrefined
cold-pressed
warm-pressed
first-pressing
virgin

(Sweet) Almond Kernel Oil

(Prunus amygdalus, P. dulcis) **Botanical Family: Rosaceae**

Skin Types Suited All, particularly: sensitive	Skin Uses		Other Light texture – easily absorbed
	dryness inflammation itching soreness wrinkles	emollient nourishing revitalising	

Contains:
Olein (main component), linoleic acid, glucosides, minerals, vitamin D. Rich in proteins.

Source:
From the kernel of the nut. Contains 50–60 per cent oil. Produced in Europe, the USA and Asia. Extracted by several methods. Often cold-pressed, then clarified.

Colour Clear pale yellow	Odour None to delicate

Directions
Can be used undiluted.

Special Note
There is an oil called 'bitter almond' (P. amara). This is considered hazardous, and is not used in aromatherapy.

Apricot Kernel Oil

(Prunus armeniaca, Armeniaca vulgaris) **Botanical Family: Rosaceae**

Skin Types Suited All, particularly: dry prematurely aged sensitive	Skin Uses		Other Light texture – easily absorbed
	dryness inflammation sensitive skins wrinkles	moisturising nourishing	

Contains:
Minerals, traces of vitamins (including vitamin B17), proteins. High in polyunsaturates and essential fatty acids.

Source:
From the kernel of the nut. Extracted by several methods.

Colour Colourless to pale yellow	Odour None to slight

Directions
Can be used undiluted.

Avocado Flesh Oil

(Persea americana, P. gratissima) Botanical Family: Lauraceae

Skin Types Suited All, particularly:	Skin Uses		Other
ageing degenerated dehydrated dry prematurely lined sensitive	eczema psoriasis	moisturising purifying restorative softening soothing	A thick oil – penetrative, easily absorbed

Contains:
Vitamins A, D, E, mineral potassium, proteins, lecithin, fatty acids. High in mono-unsaturates, chlorophyll linoleic acid.

Source:
Expressed from the flesh of the fruit, which is often dried. Contains 30 per cent oil. Extracted by hydraulic presses and centrifuge.

Colour	Odour
Light to dark, rich green (Refined oil is yellow)	Yes (Refined oil is odourless)

Directions
Generally used as an addition to the base oil, at 10 per cent of the whole. Can be used up to 30 per cent of the whole.

Borage Seed Oil

(Borago officinalis) Botanical Family: Boraginaceae

Skin Types Suited	Skin Uses		Other
dry prematurely aged inflamed lifeless mature stressed reactive types	eczema inflammation lined skin psoriasis General skin care for aged skin	emollient regenerating revitalising	Thick oil

Contains:
Vitamins, minerals and the highest amount of gamma linolenic acid (GLA).

Source:
From the seeds of the borage plant. Purchase organic, cold-pressed.

Colour	Odour
Pale golden yellow	Slight

Directions
Generally used as an addition to the base oil, at 10 per cent of the whole. Can be used up to 20 per cent of the whole.

Camellia Seed Oil		
(Camellia japonica) **Botanical Family: Theaceae**		
Skin Types Suited **All, particularly:** ageing dry normal mature sensitive	**Skin Uses** dryness *emollient* flakiness *firming* itching *moisturising* soreness *soothing* wrinkles *toning* *Good regenerative face oil*	**Other** *Slightly thick, easily absorbed*
Contains: High content of oleic acid.		
Source: From the seeds of the tree. Cultivated in Japan.		
Colour Pale yellow	**Odour** Slight	
Directions Used in blends. Can be used undiluted.		

Castor Oil		
(Ricinus communis) **Botanical Family: Euphorbiaceae**		
Skin Types Suited Body oil only	**Skin Uses** acne eczema itching psoriasis rashes	**Other** *Thick oil, waterproof and lubricating. 'Red turkey oil', which is water soluble, is sulfonated castor oil.*
Contains: Palmatic (fatty acid and others), ricinaleic acid, glycerine.		
Source: From the beans of the plant. Native to India and West Africa.		
Colour Yellow	**Odour** Slight	
Directions Generally used as an addition to body base oil, at 10 per cent of the whole.		

Coconut Oil

(Cocos nucifera) Botanical Family: Palmaceae

Skin Types Suited	Skin Uses		Other
Body oil only	stretch marks	*cleansing* *softening* *soothing*	*Mainly used as a body oil. Can cause irritation on sensitive skins*

Contains:
Palmatic (fatty acid and others), ricinaleic acid, glycerine.

Source:
Native to tropical coasts.
Can be purchased deodorised, and in this form is often used by massage therapists.

Colour	Odour
Colourless White when cold and solid	Yes No when deodorised

Directions
Use as an addition to the body base oil, at 10 per cent of the whole.

Evening Primrose Seed Oil

(Oenothera biennis) Botanical Family: Onagraceae

Skin Types Suited	Skin Uses		Other
ageing dehydrated dry flaking fragile mature menopausal prematurely aged pre-menstrual stressed	bruising eczema itching psoriasis scarring	*regenerating* *rejuvenating* *moisturising* *soothing*	*Easily absorbed, thick oil*

Contains:
Essential fatty acids, gamma lineolic acid (GLA), proteins, vitamins, minerals.

Source:
From the seeds of the plant.

Colour	Odour
Pale yellow	Slightly

Directions
Use as an addition to the base oil, up to 10 per cent of the whole.

Grapeseed Oil		
(Vitis vinifera) Botanical Family: Vitaceae		
Skin Types Suited Body skin – all	**Skin Uses** For general body work use – not recommended in face oils	**Other** Good massage oil. Stays fresh longer than many other oils
Contains: High in polyunsaturates, vitamins including F, minerals.		
Source: From the seed. Contains 6–20 per cent oil.		
Colour Unrefined – pale green Refined – pale yellow	**Odour** Slight	
Directions Can be used undiluted in body oils only.		

Hazelnut Oil			
(Corylus avellana) Botanical Family: Betulaceae			
Skin Types Suited **All, particularly:** damaged oily with dry patches sensitive	**Skin Uses** dryness wrinkles	moisturising revitalising soothing softening	**Other** Fine textured oil – easily absorbed; highly penetrative; excellent for facials
Contains: Proteins, vitamins, minerals, essential fatty acids, linolenic acid.			
Source: From the hazel kernel.			
Colour Yellow	**Odour** Slight		
Directions Can be used undiluted.			

Jojoba

(Simmondsia chinensis) Botanical Family: Buxacea

Skin Types Suited All, particularly:	Skin Uses		Other
combination inflamed: red mature oily and dry sensitive	acne eczema dryness flaking psoriasis soreness stretch marks	anti-inflammatory emollient moisturising	For general use; highly penetrative. Considered a liquid wax – similar structure to sebum

Contains:
Proteins, minerals, myristic acid and a substance that mimics collagen. Rich in vitamin E.

Source:
From the jojoba bean. South American in origin.

Colour	Odour
Pale yellow	Some

Directions
Can be used undiluted, but usually used as a 30 per cent addition to a base oil.

Macadamia Nut Oil

(Macadamia ternifolia/integrifolia) Botanical Family: Protoceae

Skin Types Suited All, particularly:	Skin Uses		Other
ageing dry mature sensitive	wrinkles	emollient rejuvenating restorative revitalising softening	A light, penetrating oil. Contains the same components found in human sebum – the only known plant to do so. Good for general skin care

Contains:
Essential fatty acid – palmifoleic acid. Vitamin A.

Source:
From nut kernel. Origin Australia.

Colour	Odour
Pale yellow	Slight

Directions
Can be used undiluted.

Passion Flower Seed Oil

(Passiflora incarnata) Botanical Family: Passifloraceae

Skin Types Suited All, particularly:	Skin Uses		Other
ageing	dryness	emollient	Fine textured oil
dry	wrinkles	rejuvenation	with good
normal	slackness	revitalisation	penetrative
mature		toning	properties
sensitive	Good for skins requiring elasticity		

Contains:
Polyunsaturated linoleic acid, high level of fatty acids. Vitamin E and minerals.

Source:
From the warmed seeds. Produced in Brazil.

Colour	Odour
Pale yellow	Rare

Directions
Can be used undiluted. Or use as an addition of 20 per cent of the whole.

Peach kernel Oil

(Prunus persica) Botanical Family: Roseaceae

Skin Types Suited All, particularly:	Skin Uses		Other
ageing	dryness	moisturising	Light oil with
dehydrated	flaking	rejuvenation	good
normal	loss of	revitalisation	penetrative
sensitive	elasticity	softening	properties; easily absorbed

Contains:
Mono- and polyunsaturates, essential fatty acids, vitamins A and E.

Source:
From the kernel of the peach nut. Produced in China.

Colour	Odour
Pale golden yellow	Slightly sweet to none

Directions
Can be used undiluted.

Rosehip Seed Oil

(Rosa rubiginosa) Botanical Family: Rosaceae

Skin Types Suited All, particularly:	Skin Uses	Other
damaged dry mature prematurely ageing sun damaged	burns mobility of tissue crow's feet rejuvenating scar tissue regenerative scarring toning wrinkles	Thick oil; often sold deodorised

Contains:
Linoleic and linolenic fatty acids, oleic acid, rich in transretinoic acid, vitamins including A, proteins, minerals.

Source:
From the seeds, by solvent extraction. Produced in Chile.

Colour	Odour
Orange/reddish gold	Yes No – deodorised

Directions
Can be used undiluted on specific areas, or diluted at 20 per cent for more general use.

Wild rose (rosehip)

Sesame Oil

(Sesamum indicum) Botanical Family: Pedaliaceae

Skin Types Suited All, particularly:	Skin Uses	Other
dehydrated dry normal sun damaged	dryness moisturising eczema nourishing flaking soothing psoriasis	

Contains:
Mono-unsaturated fatty acids, linoleic acids, proteins, minerals, calcium, magnesium, vitamins B and E, lecithin, amino acids, phosphorus, methionine.

Source:
From the seeds – 60 per cent oil. Produced in Asia and the Mediterranean.

Colour	Odour
Light golden yellow	Slight to strong

Directions
Use as an addition to the base oil, at 10 per cent of the whole.

Tamanu/Kamanu		
(Calophyllum inophyllum) Botanical Family: Guttiferaceae		
Skin Types Suited broken capillaries problem skin skin in need of repair	**Skin Uses** acne inflammation eczema scarring	**Other** Can be used on shingles
Contains: Saturated, polyunsaturated and monosaturated fatty acids.		
Source: From the fruit and seeds. Rare oil from Polynesia, East Africa, Eastern India.		
Colour Dark green	**Odour** Strong	
Directions Use as specific-area application undiluted.		

Wheatgerm Oil		
(Triticum vulgare) Botanical Family: Poaceae		
Skin Types Suited All, particularly: dry mature normal prematurely aged	**Skin Uses** eczema emollient inflamed soothing psoriasis scar tissue	**Other** Viscous sticky oil, often sold deodorised. Natural anti-oxidant. May cause irritation and sensitivity in those allergic to wheat
Contains: Richest source of vitamin E. Natural anti-oxidant. Essential fatty acids, proteins, minerals, phosphorus, zinc, iron, potassium, sulphur, rich source of vitamin E and vitamins B1, B2, B3, B6, linoleic acid.		
Source: From the germ of wheat.		
Colour Orange	**Odour** Yes	
Directions Use as an addition to the base oil, at 10 per cent of the whole.		

Infused or Macerated Oils

Calendula (Marigold)		
(Calendula officinalis) Botanical Family: Asteraceae		
Skin Types Suited Body only: chapped cracked damaged sore	**Skin Uses** chapping softening eczema soothing inflammation irritation itchiness rashes	**Other** Macerated oil
Source: From the petals of the flowers.		
Colour Yellow to orange	**Odour** Yes	
Directions Use undiluted on specific body areas, or as a 10 per cent addition to body massage oil.		

Carrot (Red) Root Extract Oil		
(Daucus carota) Botanical Family: Apiaceae		
Skin Types Suited dry mature normal oily prematurely aged problem	**Skin Uses** acne eczema anti-oxidant itching regenerating psoriasis revitalising scarring skin purifier scar tissue	**Other** Extracted from root and added to vegetable oil – consistency depends on which, generally soya
Contains: Beta carotene, vitamins A, B1, B2, C, D, E, F, minerals.		
Source: From the root		
Colour Deep red orange – varying degrees	**Odour** Slight	
Directions Use in moderation or it will dye the skin. Use as an addition to up to approximately 5 per cent of the whole.		

St. John's Wort Oil			
(Hypericum perforatum) **Botanical Family: Hypericaceae**			
Skin Types Suited Body only: chapped cracked damaged sore	**Skin Uses** bruising inflammation	*soothing*	**Other** *Macerated oil; may increase photosensitivity, not to be used before going in the sun*
Source: From the stems, leaves and flowers.			
Colour Red		**Odour** Slight	
Directions Use undiluted on specific body areas, or as a 10 per cent addition to body massage oil.			

Vegetable Oil Ingredients

Essential Fatty Acids

These are useful in beauty treatment because they help build the membranes that surround all living cells, strengthen the lipidic barrier and thus prevent the loss of moisture. A lack of essential fatty acids can show in dry skin with a lack of vitality, and a prematurely aged appearance.

Linoleic Acid

A lack of linoleic acid can contribute to premature ageing of the collagen fibres, and can be evident as hair loss, or in slow wound healing.

Vitamin E

Vitamin E helps repair collagen. A lack of vitamin E can contribute to blotchiness, a loss of firmness and skin tone, and give the impression of premature ageing. Vitamin E is needed by the body as an anti-oxidant, and to fight the occurrence of free radicals.

Vitamin D

A lack of vitamin D leads to sluggishness in cell proliferation. Skin tissue is slow to repair and there can be hyperkeratosis (the cells die before reaching the skin surface). Lack of vitamin D may be the cause of a dry flaky complexion, and other skin problems. Dandruff can also be a sign of vitamin D deficiency.

Lecithin

Lecithin is a component of cellular membranes, and is needed to metabolise blood fats.

CHAPTER 4

Essential Oils and Hydrolats

Essential oils are very concentrated liquids produced in specialist cells of certain plants. Not all plants produce essential oil, and not all essential oils found in plants are used in aromatherapy. There are around half a million plant species in the world, and aromatherapy uses essential oils from approximately one hundred. People all over the world have, over thousands of years, discovered which plants are beneficial to them and, of these, which produce essential oil in enough quantity to make extraction practical. With the development of modern, more productive distillation processes, a greater number of essential oils are becoming available.

WHERE DO ESSENTIAL OILS COME FROM, AND WHY DOES THE PLANT PRODUCE THEM?

Essential oils are produced in specialist cells of plants. Depending on the plant species, these cells are known as *glands*, *glandular hairs*, *secretory cells*, *oil ducts* and *resin ducts*. These specialist cells are thought to produce the essential oils for different reasons:

- *Reproduction*   By releasing the volatile aromatic molecules of their essential oil, the plant attracts the insects it needs to pollinate, and reproduce.
- *Protection*   (a) By releasing their aroma into the surrounding atmosphere, the essential oils act as a deterrent to insects or animals that might otherwise eat the plant. (b) Within the plant, the essential oil molecules taste unappetising to insects or animals who attempt to eat it.
- *Protection*   Being anti-bacterial, anti-viral, or anti-fungal agents, they protect the plant from micro-organisms which can damage plants in the same way as their animal-living cousins can damage humans.
- *Survival mechanism*   By acting as a reserve energy source in times of environmental stress, during drought, climatic change or after physical damage.

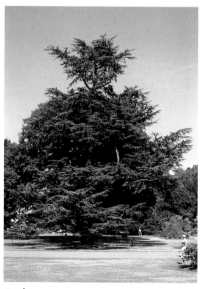

Cedar tree

Essential oils are produced in different parts of plants, depending on the species. For example:

- *Petals or whole flowers*   neroli, rose, ylang-ylang, camomile german;
- *Flowering tops*   clary sage, lavender, marjoram, yarrow;

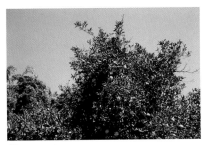
Orange tree

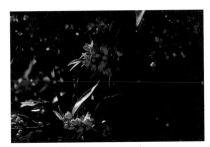
Orange blossom – neroli

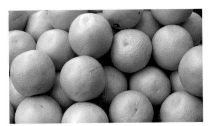
Orange fruit

- *Leaves*   geranium, violet, eucalyptus, tea tree;
- *Foliage and twigs*   cypress, petitgrain, rosemary, myrtle;
- *Over-ground whole plant*   basil, camomile maroc (ormenis), peppermint, spearmint;
- *Grasses*   lemongrass, palmarosa, gingergrass;
- *Seeds*   fennel, coriander, angelica, dill;
- *Fruits or fruit peel*   bergamot, juniper, lemon, mandarin;
- *Woods or bark*   sandalwood, cedarwood, amyris, ho-wood;
- *Rhizomes and roots*   ginger, vetiver, spikenard, valerian;
- *Resin or gum*   frankincense, myrrh, elemi, galbanham.

CHARACTERISTICS OF ESSENTIAL OILS

- Although they are called essential 'oils', the vast majority are not oily. Most essential oils have a watery **consistency**, some are slightly viscous, others are viscous.
- Essential oils are **volatile**, which means they evaporate. If a bottle of essential oil is left open, or if the essential oils are placed in a bowl or dish, they will evaporate. When subjected to heat, essential oils evaporate more quickly.
- Each essential oil has a characteristic **fragrance**, unique to the particular plant species from which it comes. The fragrance of an essential oil reflects its chemical composition.

A few plants produce more than one essential oil, and in these cases the essential oil has a fragrance characteristic of that plant-part. For example, neroli essential oil is produced from orange tree blossom, while petitgrain essential oil is produced from the twigs, stems and small unripe fruit of the orange tree. Neroli and petitgrain essential oils smell different from each other, as the essential oil is taken from two differing parts of the orange tree. Orange essential oil is extracted from the rind of the fruit.

Although an essential oil has an individual fragrance generally characteristic of the plant, there is great variation in aroma and therapeutic value even between essential oils of the same species. These differences depend on the geographical location in which the plant was grown, the cultivation conditions, at what time of year and time of day the plant was harvested, and the extraction procedures. Variations occur owing to:

- the soil in which the plant is grown (country, or location in country), nutrients in the soil, pesticides, herbicides and fertilisers used;
- altitude at which grown;
- weather conditions during growing season – amount of rain or sunlight;
- time of year harvested (may be two crops per year);
- time of day when the crop is harvested (before dawn or early evening, for example);
- pre-extraction preparation (chopping or crushing, for example);
- whether plant material is distilled fresh or dry;
- extraction process chosen;

- heat and length of distillation;
- care in handling after extraction;
- storage history – age of oil.

'NOTES' – THE PERFUMER'S ART

Essential oils were once the mainstay of perfumery, and are still included in some of the most exclusive perfumes. Aromatherapy has adopted the perfumer's vocabulary of 'notes'. The rate at which an aroma, or chemical component of an aroma, evaporates determines whether it is 'top note' (evaporates quickly), 'middle note' (evaporates at an average rate) or 'base note' (evaporates slowly).

An important aspect of the perfumer's art is to create a perfume so that the fragrance remains beautiful at all stages – when first put on the skin, shortly after, and later in the day. In the same way, when blending essential oils to create a pleasant aroma for non-therapeutic purposes, essential oils can be blended with these notes in mind.

A particular essential oil can fall into two groups, depending on the other essential oils it is blended with. For example, geranium oil may be a top note in one blend, but act as a middle note in another blend which includes an essential oil that is more highly volatile. The difference in category is a matter of relativity: in the first blend, geranium is considered the top note because it is *relatively* more volatile than the other ingredients; but becomes a middle note in the second blend because it is *relatively* less volatile than the other ingredients. Consequently, geranium and other oils may be defined as 'top-to-middle' notes. The note of each essential oil is given in their individual profiles later in this chapter.

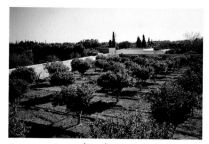
Orange (neroli) plantation, Tunisia

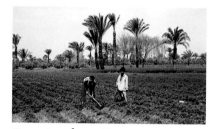
Geranium farm, Egypt

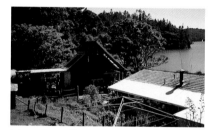
Manuka still, New Zealand

PHYSICAL VARIATION

Essential oils vary in their physical characteristics, in terms of their:

- colour
- viscosity

In addition, certain oils change consistency according to their

- temperature

Colour

Essential oils are differently coloured:

- Many are colourless (eucalyptus radiata, lavender, rosemary) or have a slight yellow or green tinge (bergamot, geranium, cypress, melissa). Some fall within the stronger colour range of yellow–orange–brown (mandarin, patchouli, myrrh), while others are blue owing to the azulene content of the oil (camomile german, yarrow).

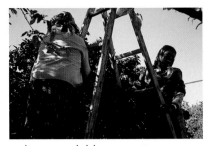

Picking neroli blossoms, Tunisia

USEFUL DILUTED OILS
Orange Blossom (Neroli), Rose, Jasmine

- The colour of an essential oil can change over time.
- Variations in colour can be detected from year to year, and from county to country of production.

Viscosity

Most essential oils are very fluid (black pepper, camomile roman, cypress, eucalyptus radiata, fennel, juniper, lavender, neroli, peppermint, petitgrain, rosemary, tea tree), others can be less fluid (camomile german, jasmine, ylang-ylang, cedarwood), while a few are viscous – which means they are thicker in consistency (sandalwood, vetiver, myrrh).

Temperature

Some essential oils become solid when in cooler temperatures. For example, rose otto changes to a solid, crystalline consistency (see *Storage* in Chapter 6), others become thicker when subjected to heat – for example, myrrh and vetiver.

STARTER KIT

ESSENTIAL OILS STARTER KIT
Lavender, Geranium, Sandalwood, Camomile Roman, Lemon, Palmarosa, Petitgrain, Rosemary, Ylang-ylang, Tea Tree

Throughout the book you will find essential oil advice for all the specific skin types and conditions, many of which will require the use of essential oils not listed here. But as a 'starter kit', all the essential oils listed could be used for beauty therapy purposes. The essential oils listed are reasonable in price. As a next step, the following three essential oils could be included in the beauty therapist's kit. These more expensive essential oils and absolutes can often be purchased already diluted.

HOW ESSENTIAL OILS ARE EXTRACTED FROM PLANTS

The method chosen to extract an essential oil depends on the type of plant material in which that oil is found. For example, jasmine flowers are too delicate to survive the heat of steam distillation, and their essential oil has traditionally been extracted by a method that does not involve heat, called *enfleurage*. This is a much more time-consuming method and involves laying the petals in fat which absorbs the essential oil. The essential oil is later separated from the fat, although today Jasmine is more likely to be extracted by solvent.

The main methods of essential oil extraction are:

- *steam distillation*
- *dry steam distillation*
- *hydrodiffusion*
- *enfleurage*
- *maceration*
- *expression*
- *solvent extraction*

Steam Distillation

Steam distillation is by far the most common method of essential oil extraction. The plant material is placed in a still, along with a larger volume of water. It is heated to boiling, and the steam evaporates. In that steam are molecules of essential oil, which have been released from the plant material by the heating process. The steam and essential oil molecules rise, and enter a pipe known as a 'gooseneck', which leads to a second chamber containing a downward-running coiled pipe. This is cooled by refrigerated water in the second chamber, a process that returns the steam to liquid. This liquid contains both the condensed water vapour and the essential oil – which have a different density from each other, and thus separate. The essential oil can then easily be siphoned off.

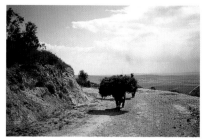
Carrying the crop – wild rosemary

Dry Steam Distillation

This method is technically very similar to steam distillation, except that the plant material is not placed in water. Instead, it is put on a grate within the still, and is subjected to highly heated steam. Under pressure from this heated steam, the essential oil-bearing plant cells expand, releasing their essential oil, which joins the steam vapour. As with steam distillation, the steam is cooled by running through the refrigerated coil, the condensed water and essential oil separate, and the essential oil is siphoned off.

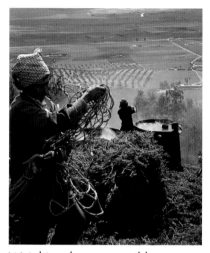
Weighing the crop – wild rosemary

Hydrodiffusion

Hydrodiffusion differs from steam distillation only in that the steam enters at the top of the still, above the plant material, rather than below it. Hydrodiffusion is very well suited to wood or fibrous material, as the steam can percolate through it.

Enfleurage

Some flowers do not respond well to heat, so the essential oil must be extracted using some other method. Enfleurage is an ancient method, and very labour intensive. It involves laying the flowers, one by one, on sheets of glass, each covered with a thick layer of odourless fat. When ready, several layers are sealed within a wooden frame. The fat absorbs the essential oil from the flower petals. After a period of time, the flowers are replaced. Jasmine is replaced after 24 hours, tuberose after 72 hours. It takes around a month of constantly replacing the flowers in this way before the fat is sufficiently saturated with the essential oil. At this stage the fat it known as *pomade*. Unheated alcohol is used to separate the essential oil from the fat. This method can only be used with flowers that remain fragrant for some time after picking.

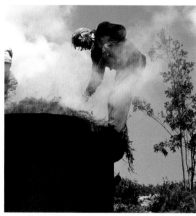
Distilling the crop – wild rosemary

Maceration

Maceration is a method sometimes used with flowers that lose their fragrance – their essential oil – almost immediately after picking. The flowers are placed in oil or fat which is gently heated to 60–70°C, thus breaking down the essential oil-bearing cells. The essential oil is absorbed into the oil or fat. Plant material is put in the oil or fat for about an hour, and the process is repeated around a dozen times, before the oil or fat is separated from the essential oil.

Expression

The citrus essential oils, such as lemon, lime, bergamot, grapefruit, mandarin, tangerine, and yuzu, are contained in the fruit peel – the zest. In historic times the essential oil was extracted by continuously pressing natural sponges into the rind and then squeezing them out. Today the oil is extracted by piercing or scratching the peel mechanically, or by crushing it between rollers. The essential oil can then be separated from the pith by spinning the mixed pulp in a centrifuge machine.

Solvent Extraction

This is the most modern of the extraction methods and involves using various chemicals as solvents. The solvent must boil at a low heat so that the essential oils are not damaged, and must be completely evaporated so that no residue is left. This method produces a semi-solid mass, called a *concrete*, which can be further treated with alcohol to produce an *absolute* – which is a highly concentrated form of essential oil.

Liquid carbon dioxide (CO_2) is the most recent addition to the solvents used in extraction, and has made it possible to extract essential oils from lilac and other plants, which was not possible before. CO_2-extracted oils have different properties from other essential oils, as they contain compounds from all the plant material, both the lighter and heavier elements.

HYDROLATS – AROMATIC HYDROSOLS

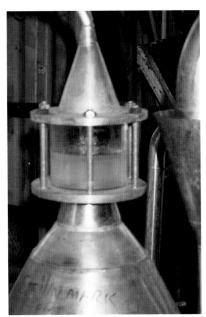

Hydrolat shown under essential oil layer in flask

- Hydrolats are extremely valuable as beauty therapy products, and can be used on their own as tonics, or in compresses, or incorporated into masks.
- Hydrolats are a by-product of essential oil production. During distillation, the essential oil is separated from the water or condensed steam used in the process. The remaining water is impregnated with the hydrophilic (water-soluble) compounds of the essential oil, and is known as the hydrolat (or aromatic hydrosol).
- As the water used in distillation is imbued only with the water-soluble components of essential oils, hydrolats cannot be considered as 'watered down essential oils'. Although both hydrolats and essential oils come from the same plant material, they each contain components not present in the other. Hydrolats are therefore an additional beauty therapy tool.

- The best known hydrolat is 'rose-water', which is used in many countries as an ingredient in cooking. However, this product has usually been diluted many times before it reaches the retail stage and often contains preservatives.
- In beauty therapy, pure hydrolats should be purchased from professional aromatherapy suppliers, or from medical herbalism suppliers – as hydrolats such as rosemary, thyme, lavender, tea tree and camomile are used in medical herbalism.
- Hydrolats are very gentle, and useful in cases where essential oils may be considered too strong. However, they are also very effective in treatments for most skin types, as outlined in the following chart.

HYDROLATS AND THEIR USES

	Angelica seed	Calendula	Camomile german	Camomile roman	Carrot seed	Cedarwood	Clary sage	Eucalyptus	Fennel	Helichrysum	Laurel	Lavender	Linden blossom	Melissa	Myrtle	Neroli	Peppermint	Rose	Rosemary	Sage	Thyme	Verbena	Yarrow
Most skins	★		★	★								★				★		★				★	
Normal skin	★		★	★	★		★		★			★				★						★	
Sensitive skin			★	★								★	★	★		★		★					
Dry skin			★	★					★			★		★				★		★			
Oily skin	★	★				★	★	★				★			★				★		★	★	★
Ageing skin			★	★	★		★			★	★	★				★		★		★			
Sluggish skin	★	★					★	★						★	★	★	★	★		★			
Tonic									★	★						★	★	★	★				
Astringent						★		★			★					★						★	★
Stimulating							★				★						★	★					
Refreshing					★			★	★			★		★		★	★	★	★				
Regenerative			★	★	★					★		★	★	★	★			★	★	★			
Balancing	★		★	★			★					★			★			★		★	★		
Soothing			★	★					★			★	★		★	★							
Softening	★								★					★		★		★					
Acne and spots		★	★	★		★	★	★		★	★	★		★					★				★
Skin infections						★	★			★	★								★	★			
Inflammation			★	★								★											★
Eczema and psoriasis			★	★					★			★											★
Scars				★						★		★				★		★		★			★
Sore eyes *(pads on closed eyelids only)*		★	★	★			★		★			★				★		★				★	

MAKING ESSENTIAL OIL 'WATERS'

Essential oil teas are made in the following way:

- add 3 ml (¹/₁₀th ounce) of essential oil to each litre of water, boiling on a cooker;
- cover the pot with a lid;
- allow to simmer for 10 minutes;
- allow to cool with the lid in place;
- pour through an unbleached paper coffee filter;
- bottle for future use.

MAKING HERBAL 'TEAS'

Use the same method as above, but instead of essential oil use either:

113.4 grams (4 ounces) of dried herb

or

226.8 grams (8 ounces) of fresh herb

to each litre (2.1 pints) of water.

ESSENTIAL OIL 'WATERS'

Essential oil 'waters' are water infused with essential oil. They are not hydrolats, because they do not contain the hydrophilic compounds that become infused in the water used in the distillation process. Nor are they watered down essential oils because the action of boiling the water, and of filtering it through paper, removes some of the essential oil components.

Essential oil 'waters' can be used in the following ways: compresses, saunas, steam rooms, baths and as an ingredient in beauty products. They are *not* a substitute for hydrolats, although they can be used in this way as herbal 'teas'.

THE CHEMISTRY OF ESSENTIAL OILS

Essential oils are a very complex mix of naturally occurring aromatic chemicals, known as its *components*. Identifying which chemicals exist in any one essential oil is not an easy task because as well as the approximately 30000 known aromatic molecules, there are many as yet unidentified components. On average, each essential oil is made up of between 100 and 300 components, although some contain fewer and some contain more.

Each of the components has its own aroma and potential therapeutic action, and the unique character of each whole essential oil is determined by the particular mix of components and their relative amounts. Sometimes the compounds present in minute quantity have an important role. For example, rose oil contains 300 components, yet it derives its distinctive aroma from β-damascenone, which is only 0.14 per cent of the whole.

By looking at the main chemical groups of an essential oil, one can make a fair judgement as to whether that oil can perform a particular task. For example, if looking for an essential oil that can be used to fight bacteria, those containing large amounts of phenols and monoterpenes would be possible options. Then one might need to consider whether treatment should be more powerful and short-term (phenols), or less powerful and long-term (monoterpenes).

On the other hand, if the essential oil is being chosen for its relaxing effect, a more appropriate mixture of chemicals within the essential oil would include larger amounts of the aldehydes, coumarins, ethers, esters, lactones and sesquiterpenes. However, this is not to say that choosing essential oils is a simple matter of chemical analysis, because the essential oils are extremely complex and often defy the rules. For example, geranium essential oil is known to perform certain tasks, yet these are not easily attributed to its known ingredients.

There is nothing simplistic about essential oils, because they contain many trace compounds – very small components, some of which may not even have been analysed scientifically. It is the whole cocktail – *all* the ingredients – that make an essential oil what it is.

When looking at the aromatic compounds of an essential oil for its possible harmful effects, the same complications apply. Tests have shown that sensitisation occurs when certain isolated aldehydes were applied on skin; yet when these same aldehydes were applied when still within the whole essential oil – even at concentrations as high as 85 per cent – skin sensitisation did not occur. It was the other 15 per cent of trace compounds in the natural oil that neutralised the sensitising effect of the 85 per cent of aldehydes contained in them.

Nevertheless, chemical analysis of essential oils does hold some clues as to their efficacy with regard to particular conditions. For example, essential oils containing azulene or bisabol are known to have an anti-inflammatory effect, and this can be used in cases of inflammation.

Essential oil components are categorised both in terms of the aromatic chemicals they contain and of the chemical groups these belong to. The following chart shows the main groups, with just a few examples of the components contained in them, and their potential action.

AROMATIC CHEMICAL GROUPS, AND THEIR USES

Chemical Group	Well-being Effects	Examples
Alcohols	energising/stimulating toning/general tonic hypotensive/balancing	borneol, citronellol, geraniol, linalol, menthol, sabinol, α-terpineol, terpineol-4, thuyanol
Aldehydes	calming/relaxing sedative/hypnotic cooling/soothing	benzaldehyde, cinnamic aldehyde, citral, citronellal, geranial, myrtenal, phellandral, α-santalene
Coumarins	calming/relaxing sedative/hypnotic hypotensive	angelicine, bergaptene, citronene, furocoumarin, myristicine
Esters	anti-spasmodic/hypotensive calming/relaxing balancing/general tonic cooling/soothing	citronellyl formate, geranyl acetate, geranyl tiglate, linalyl acetate
Ethers	anti-spasmodic balancing/relaxing calming/soothing	apiol, cedryl methyl ether, methyl chavicol, methyl eugenol, myristicin, neryl acetate, transanethole
Ketones*	stimulating/warming	atlantone, camphor, carvone, cryptone, fenchone, isomenthone, jasmone, menthone, piperitone, pulegone, thujone, verbenone, vetivone
Monoterpenes	general tonic/stimulating	camphene, p-cymene, limonene, myrcene, phellandrene, α- and β-pinene, sabinene, α-, γ- and g-terpinene, thujene
Oxides	stimulating/warming	bisabolol oxide, bisabolone oxide, 1,8-cineole, linalol oxide, piperitonoxide, rose oxide
Phenols*	stimulating/warming	australol, carvacrol, chavicol, eugenol, gaiacol, thymol, anethole, cinnamaldehyde, estragol
Sesquiterpenes	calming/relaxing general tonic/anti-spasmodic anti-inflammatory anti-allergenic	bisabolol, carotol, β-caryophyllene, chamazulene, β-eudesmol, farnesol, patchouline, α-santalol, zingiberol

*Essential oils with a high percentage of this group of chemicals are often contra-indicated in aromatherapy (refer to list in Chapter 6); others are not.

ADULTERATION OF ESSENTIAL OILS AND THE IMPORTANCE OF PURITY

For many years the essential oils produced in the world were destined for the perfume and flavour industries and, today, many of the recommendations regarding the use of essential oils reflect a concern with *fragrance*, *taste* and *shelf-life*, rather than with *therapeutic value*. Industry is also more concerned with consistency of product and price. For all these reasons, you have to be very careful that the product you buy has not been adulterated in some way.

These are some of the ways in which essential oils can be manipulated:

Nature-identicals

In some cases, a component is added to the essential oil. Nature-identicals are naturally occurring chemicals that have been extracted from plants – either from other varieties of the plant from which the essential oil is derived or from unrelated species of plants. Nature-identicals are components that already exist in the essential oil they are being added to. They are added for two reasons:

- To add volume to the essential oil, making it go further, financially speaking, for the producer.
- To bring the essential oil within guidelines. Certain standards are set, stating that an essential oil must contain a precise amount of a particular chemical. But sometimes a particular batch of essential oil does not contain the required amount of the chemical – either because of growing conditions in that particular year, or as a result of errors in the distillation process. Producers thus add nature-identicals to the batch of essential oil so it will pass the requirements set down by testing authorities. For example, the regulations require that lavender essential oil contains 25–45 per cent linalyl acetate and 25–38 per cent linalol. If the natural oil falls outside these requirements, nature-identicals may be added.

In some cases, a so-called 'essential oil' will be a collection of nature-identical chemical components, put together to mimic a true essential oil. These products cannot perform the therapeutic tasks of true essential oils, as they lack the components that occur in the essential oils in such minute quantities they cannot be identified by chemical analysis, or are as yet unidentified by scientific means and are unnamed.

Synthetics

Synthetics do not derive from plant material, but from chemical building-blocks. They are chemically manufactured to mimic naturally occurring chemicals, and are often extended by additions of solvents. In some cases, a natural essential oil is adulterated with a synthetic additive. Geranium oil, especially the prized 'Geranium Bourbon', is sometimes adulterated in this way, making a trustworthy source essential.

In other cases, an entire so-called 'essential oil' may be a collection of synthetic chemicals, and will be totally devoid of any therapeutic value (even if the fragrance is a fair copy of the real thing).

Substitution

When an essential oil is very expensive, or in short supply, there is a risk that it may be mixed with a cheaper, or more readily available essential oil. Here are some examples of essential oils which are vulnerable to such part-substitution:

Essential Oil		Substitute Essential Oil
Fennel (sweet)	–	fennel (bitter)
Geranium	–	citronella; palmarosa
Juniper berry	–	juniper wood;
Melissa	–	lemongrass; citronella; 'melissa-like'
Neroli	–	petitgrain
Peppermint	–	cornmint
Rose maroc	–	palmarosa; geranium; citronella
Rose otto	–	palmarosa
Sandalwood	–	amyris; cedarwood
Tea tree	–	other *Melaleuca* species
Ylang-ylang	–	cananga

Rectification

Essential oils are used for many purposes other than just for aromatherapy. Some oils are used in mechanical industries, as well as for perfumes, cosmetics, foods, drinks and confectionery. These purchasers of essential oils have different requirements for their oils than do aromatherapy users, and sometimes require that certain components are removed. This is often done to make the oils last longer, or to be more soluble in alcohol, or comply with certain regulations. Such manipulated oils do not have the therapeutic qualities attributed to them by aromatherapy knowledge, but can still find their way to the aromatherapy market.

Mixing

Different batches of the same essential oil are mixed together. Sometimes the oils are mixed in this way to disguise age, quality or aroma. By mixing, the manufacturer hopes to disguise the lack of quality of the product.

Dilution

The essential oil is diluted. If it has been diluted in a vegetable oil, that is easy to detect, as it will leave an oily residue on a piece of paper (whereas pure essential oil will usually evaporate). However, if the essential oil has been diluted with an alcohol or solvent, that is more difficult to detect.

High-priced essential oils such as rose, jasmine, hyacinth, carnation and tuberose are often sold diluted in a fixed oil such as jojoba, so as to allow therapists to experience them without incurring such high costs as would be encountered when purchasing them undiluted. This is perfectly acceptable, so long as the product is marketed and labelled as being diluted.

ENSURING PURITY

Essential oils are adulterated because demand outstrips supply. The best judge of purity is not a machine – which can be fooled by adulteration by both nature-identicals and synthetics – but a human nose. However, it takes time to develop the skills required to distinguish between good-quality oils and adulterated oils.

To help ensure purity, the following steps could be followed:

- take every opportunity to compare by smell different essential oils from a variety of suppliers;
- purchase from suppliers who provide the botanical species of the plant that the essential oil has been extracted from, and the country of origin;
- ask your supplier if their oils have been analysed by gas chromatography combined with mass spectrometry.

QUALITY TESTING OF ESSENTIAL OILS

Essential oils are tested by their physical characteristics, and their chemical components. The physical tests consist of:

- *specific density* – their weight;
- *optical rotation* – whether they bend polarised light clockwise (+) or anticlockwise (–), as measured by a polarimeter;
- *refractive index* – the speed at which light passes through it;
- *solubility in alcohol*.

Specific tests can be carried out to identify the presence of alcohols, esters, aldehydes and ketones, but more usually the chemical constituents of essential oils are tested by:

- *Gas chromatography (GC)* – the essential oil is heated and vaporised, and carried by hydrogen gas through a column packed with inert matter coated with a non-volatile liquid phase. The column is contained in an oven, which heats it from 70° to 270°C (158° to 518°F), rising at 2°C (36°F) every minute. As the components of essential oils evaporate at different rates, they can be identified as they reach the end of the column, by means of a flame ionisation detector, and recorded on a graph – the GC 'fingerprint' of an essential oil.
- *Mass spectrometry* – the essential oil is bombarded with electrons, breaking apart the molecules. As each chemical fragments in a pattern unique to itself, the components of the essential oil can be identified.

THE ESSENTIAL OIL BEAUTY PROFILES

Beauty therapy is concerned with the therapeutic action of essential oils as they affect the physical appearance of the face

TIP

HOW TO EVALUATE THE SMELL OF AN ESSENTIAL OIL
- Use a paper smelling strip
- Return to re-smell the essential oil several times, over a period of at least 24 hours
- Only evaluate a maximum of two essential oils each time

and body. Beauty is, of course, more than skin deep, and a person's overall physical and emotional health has a tremendous bearing on their looks. Although essential oils do have many properties that have a direct bearing on physical and emotional well-being, they are not the subject of this book, and are not included in the following profiles. If you wish to acquire greater understanding of the medicinal action of essential oils, please refer to the titles in *Further Reading* in the Appendix at the end of this book.

Essential oils are unique among therapeutic tools in being volatile – that is, they move through the air. Because of this, they are inhaled during beauty treatments, and the client has the benefit of their well-being potential. Clients are the first to comment on this, often saying that aesthetic aromatherapy treatment has greatly improved their sense of well-being as well as their looks.

TIP

It is crucial that a beauty therapist strives to use the best organic products available. The better the quality of an essential oil, the more effective it will be in treatment.

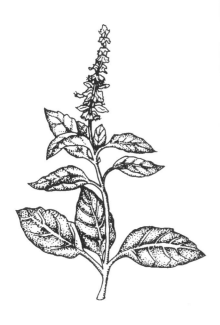

Basil (Sweet)

(Ocimum basilicum) Botanical Family: Labiatae

Herb growing up to 1 metre, with small white or pink flowers.
Plant Part used: leaves and flowering tops
Method of Extraction: steam distillation
Countries of Production: Egypt, France, USA, Bulgaria, Hungary
Fragrance: warm, aniseed-like, peppery, like the herb
Note: top to middle
Main Chemical Components:
Great variation between 'sweet' and 'exotic' types
Sweet: linalol, methyl chavicol, 1,8-cineole, eugenol, limonene
General Effect: strengthening, calming

Indicated for:

The Face	The Body
Not to be used in facial treatments	*Only to be used in low dilution* circulation stimulating congestion fatigue general aches nervous conditions stimulating tonic

Body Blending Guide:
Bergamot, black pepper, clary sage, coriander, eucalyptus, fennel, geranium, ginger, juniper, lavender, lemon, marjoram, orange, rosemary, thyme linalol

Contra-indications: *Avoid 'exotic' basil as it contains a high proportion of methyl chavicol which could cause irritation or sensitisation in some cases.* Can cause skin irritation – use with care. Avoid use in water-immersion methods unless diluted. To be avoided during pregnancy and lactation. To be avoided by those with epilepsy.	**Purchasing Guide:** **Price Range:** medium

Bergamot

(Citrus aurantium, ssp bergamia) Botanical Family: *Rutaceae*

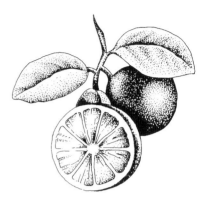

A citrus fruit tree growing up to 5 metres. Produces white, star-shaped flowers and citrus fruits that are green, becoming yellow, and the size of oranges.

Plant Part used: fruit rind
Method of extraction: cold expression
Countries of Production: Calabria/Italy, Sicily/Italy
Fragrance: rich, deep, slightly floral citrus
Note: top
Main Chemical Components:
limonene, linalyl acetate, linalol, ß-pinene, bergaptene
General Effect: refreshing, balancing

Indicated for:

The Face	The Body
Only use bergamot FCF (furocoumarin free – not phototoxic) acne blemishes infections oily skin seborrhea	*Only use bergamot FCF (furocoumarin free – not phototoxic)* acne anxiety depression psoriasis relaxing scarring stress tension

Body Blending Guide: *Suits most essential oils, including:*
Black pepper, clary sage, cypress, frankincense, geranium, jasmine, lavender, mandarin, orange, palmarosa, rosemary, vetiver, ylang-ylang

Contra-indications:	**Purchasing Guide:**
Should not be applied prior to sunbed use, or before going in prolonged sunlight	**Price Range:** medium

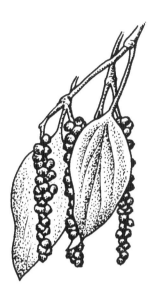

Black Pepper

(Piper nigrum) Botanical Family: Piperaceae

A woody, tree-climbing vine with strong, woody stems, small white flowers, and red berries.
Plant Part used: unripe berry
Method of Extraction: steam distillation
Countries of Production: India, China, Indonesia
Fragrance: warm and peppery, like the peppercorn
Note: middle
Main Chemical Components:
limonene, caryophyllene, α-phellandrene, α-pinene, ß-pinene
General Effect: warming, strengthening

Indicated for:

The Face	The Body
Not to be used in facial treatments	aches and pains
	circulation stimulating
	congestion
	digestion
	exhaustion
	fatigue
	muscle tone
	stiffness
	stimulating

Body Blending Guide:
Bergamot, frankincense, geranium, ginger, grapefruit, lavender, lemon, lemongrass, mandarin, marjoram, orange, palmarosa, patchouli, rosemary, sandalwood, tea tree, ylang-ylang

Contra-indications:	**Purchasing Guide:**
Can cause skin irritation – use with care. To be avoided during pregnancy and lactation.	**Price Range:** medium

Bois de Rose (Rosewood)

(Aniba rosaeodora) Botanical Family: *Lauraceae*

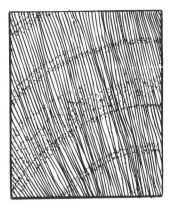

Evergreen tree native to South America, with distinctive reddish-bark.
Plant Part used: wood
Method of Extraction: steam distillation
Countries of Production: Brazil, Guiana, Peru
Fragrance: floral, woody
Note: middle
Main Chemical Components:
linalol, α-terpineol, geraniol, 1,8-cineole
General Effect: calming, balancing

Indicated for:

The Face	The Body
ageing skin	anxiety
broken capillaries	balancing
dry skin	calming
inflammation	pre-menstrual tension
itching	relaxing
mature skin	skin revitalising
normal skin	stress
revitalisation	tension
scars	
sensitive skin	
tissue regenerator	

Body Blending Guide:
Bergamot, frankincense, geranium, lavender, mandarin, neroli, orange, palmarosa, petitgrain, rose otto, tangerine, sandalwood, violet leaf, ylang-ylang

Contra-indications:
None known

Purchasing Guide:
Price Range: middle

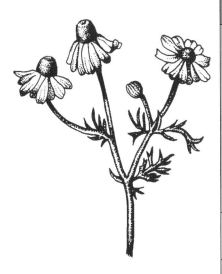

Camomile German

(Matricaria chamomilla/recutita) Botanical Family: *Asteraceae (Compositae)*

Herbaceous plant, a metre high, producing white flowers with yellow, conical-shaped centres.

Plant Part used: flowering tops
Method of Extraction: steam distillation
Countries of Production: Egypt, Hungary, Bulgaria
Fragrance: herby, hay-like
Note: middle
Main Chemical Components:
α-bisabolol, bisabolone oxide A, bisobolol oxide A, chamazulene, bisabolol B
General Effect: soothing

Indicated for:

The Face	The Body
acne	acne
broken capillaries	allergic responses
chemically damaged skin	boils
dry skin	eczema
eczema	inflammation
flaky skin	itching
infections	psoriasis
inflamed skin	rashes
itching	scarring
normal skin	spasm
psoriasis	
rashes	
redness	
scarring	
sensitive skin	

Body Blending Guide:
Bergamot, camomile roman, geranium, lavender, lemon, marjoram, niaouli, ravensara, rosemary, tea tree

Contra-indications:
None known

Purchasing Guide:
Price Range: high

Camomile Roman

(Anthemis nobilis) Botanical Family: *Asteraceae*

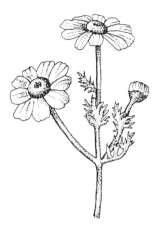

Plant growing to half a metre high, with strong stems, feathery leaves and small white flowers with yellow centres.
Plant Part used: flowers
Method of Extraction: steam distillation
Countries of Production: England, Bulgaria, Hungary, Chile
Fragrance: fruity, sweet, fresh, herby
Note: top to middle
Main Chemical Components:
α-pinene, butylangelate, 1,8-cineol, sabinene, β-pinene
General Effect: relaxing, balancing

Indicated for:

The Face	The Body
acne	aches
blemishes	anxiety
broken capillaries	calming
combination skin	insomnia
congested skin	itching
dry skin	nervous conditions
infections	pre-menstrual tension
inflammation	psoriasis
normal skin	relaxing
oily skin	skin revitalisation
rashes	soreness
sensitive skin	stiffness
	stress
	tension

Body Blending Guide:
Bergamot, clary sage, geranium, grapefruit, jasmine, lavender, lemon, mandarin, neroli, orange, palmarosa, rose otto

Contra-indications:	**Purchasing Guide:**
None known	**Price Range:** high

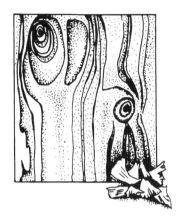

Cedarwood

(Cedrus atlantica) Botanical Family: Pinaceae

Tall evergreen tree.
Plant Part used: wood chips and sawdust
Method of Extraction: steam distillation
Countries of Production: Morocco, Algeria
Fragrance: sweet, balsamic, woody
Note: middle to base
Main Chemical Components:
cedrol, cadinene, caryophyllene, altlantone, β-cedrene
General Effect: strengthening, relaxing

Indicated for:

The Face	The Body
acne	anxiety
broken capillaries	circulation stimulating
combination skin	congestion
eczema	eczema
itching	exhaustion
normal skin	fatigue
oily skin	itching
open pores	psoriasis
rashes	rashes
seborrhoea	stressed conditions
sluggishness	tension

Body Blending Guide:
Bergamot, camomile german, camomile roman, clary sage, cypress, eucalyptus, frankincense, geranium, juniper, lavender, marjoram, orange, patchouli, petitgrain, rosemary, sandalwood, vetiver, ylang-ylang

Contra-indications:
To be avoided during pregnancy and lactation

Purchasing Guide:
There are several different types of cedarwood, but the indications above apply only to Cedrus altantica
Price Range: low

Clary Sage

(Salvia sclarea) Botanical Family: Lamiaceae (or Labiatae)

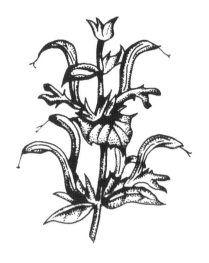

Plant growing a metre high, with lilac and pink flowers that come directly off the stem, and large, hairy leaves that grow to only half the height of the plant.

Plant Part used: flowering tops
Method of Extraction: steam distillation
Countries of Production: France, Bulgaria, Russia, Morocco
Fragrance: nutty, musty, herby
Note: middle
Main Chemical Components:
linalyl acetate, linalol, germacrene D, sclareol
General Effect: calming, balancing

Indicated for:

The Face	The Body
ageing skin	aches and stiffness
congested skin	anxiety
dry skin	depression
mature skin	dysmenorrhoea
normal skin	menopausal conditions
problem skin	nervousness
	pre-menstrual tension
	relaxing
	tension
	spasm
	stress

Blending Guide:

Bergamot, black pepper, camomile roman, geranium, grapefruit, juniper, lavender, lemon, mandarin, orange, tea tree, ylang-ylang

Contra-indications:	Purchasing Guide:
To be avoided during pregnancy and lactation	Price Range: medium

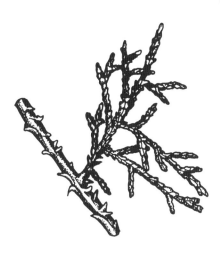

Cypress

(Cupressus sempervirens) Botanical Family: *Cupressaceae*

Evergreen cone-shaped tree growing to 7 metres. It has dark green foliage, and cones containing seed-nuts.
Plant Part used: foliage, twigs and cones of young branches;
Method of Extraction: steam distillation
Countries of Production: France, Spain, Algeria
Fragrance: fresh, woody, slightly spicy
Note: middle
Main Chemical Components:
δ−3-carene, α-pinene, terpinolene, cedrol
General Effect: stimulating, strengthening

Indicated for:

The Face	The Body
acne	astringent
broken capillaries	cellulite
combination skin	circulation stimulating
congestion	congestion
dilated pores	diuretic
improves skin tone	dysmenorrhoea
oily skin	menopause
seborrhoea	stimulating
	toning
	varicose veins

Body Blending Guide:
Bergamot, camomile german, cedarwood, clary sage, eucalyptus, frankincense, geranium, juniper, lavender, lemon, marjoram, pine, ravensara, rosemary, sandalwood, tea tree

Contra-indications:
None known

Purchasing Guide:
Price Range: medium

Eucalyptus Radiata

(Eucalyptus radiata) Botanical Family: *Myrtaceae*

A tall tree with 6-inch lance-shaped leaves, and flowers growing from a flat-topped calyx.

Plant Part used: leaves and twigs
Method of Extraction: steam distillation
Country of Production: Australia
Fragrance: woody, camphorous, medicinal
Note: top
Main Chemical Components:
1,8-cineole, α-pinene, limonene, p-cymene, α-terpineol
General Effect: invigorating, refreshing

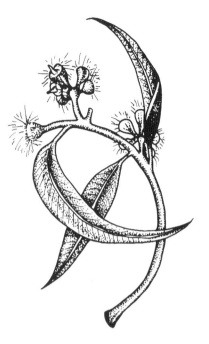

Indicated for:

The Face	The Body
Rarely used in facial treatments, except in steaming acne facial congestion oily skin sinus conditions sluggishness skin infections	aches breathing difficulties cellulite congestion inflammation itching rashes toning sluggishness stiffness stimulating

Body Blending Guide:
Camomile german, cypress, frankincense, geranium, ginger, grapefruit, juniper, lavender, lemon, marjoram, niaouli, peppermint, pine, ravensara, rosemary, tea tree, thyme linalol

Contra-indications:	**Purchasing Guide:**
Avoid using in water-immersion methods unless diluted	**Price Range:** low

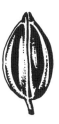

Fennel (Sweet)

(Foeniculum vulgare dulce) Botanical Family: Umbelliferae

Biennial plant growing to 2 metres, with bright green lace-like leaves, thin stalks and yellow flowers.
Plant Part used: seeds
Method of Extraction: steam distillation
Countries of Production: Spain, France, Hungary, Russia
Fragrance: sweet, aniseed-like
Note: middle to top
Main Chemical Components:
trans-anethole, fenchone, methyl chavicol, α-pinene
General Effect: energising

Indicated for:

The Face	The Body
combination skin	cellulite
mature skin	detoxifying
normal skin	digestive problems
oily skin	dysmenorrhoea
revitalising	fluid retention
toning	menopausal problems
	relaxing
	scarring
	toning

Body Blending Guide:
Basil, bergamot, black pepper, clary sage, cypress, geranium, ginger, grapefruit, juniper, lavender, lemon, marjoram, pine, rosemary, sandalwood

Contra-indications:
Can cause skin irritation – use with care.
To be avoided during pregnancy and lactation.
To be avoided by those with epilepsy.

Purchasing Guide:
Price Range: low

Frankincense

(Boswellia carterii) Botanical Family: Burseraceae

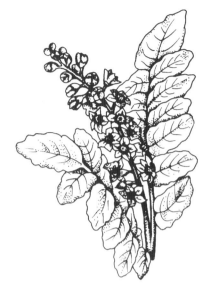

A thorny shrub. The bark produces a milky fluid which hardens on contact with the air, turning into hard, light, resin.

Plant Part used: oleoresin
Method of Extraction: steam distillation
Countries of Production: Oman, Somalia
Fragrance: warm, balsamic, incense-like
Note: middle to base
Main Chemical Components:
octyl acetate, n-octanol, α-pinene, incensyl acetate, 2, 4-incensole
General Effect: calming, soothing

Indicated for:

The Face	The Body
ageing skin	anxiety
blemishes	breathing problems
combination skin	congestion
congestion	depression
flaking skin	exhaustion
infections	scarring
mature skin	skin infections
oily skin	stress conditions
revitalisation	tension
scarring	
sinus problems	
sluggishness	

Body Blending Guide:
Bergamot, bois de rose, clary sage, geranium, jasmine, lavender, lemon, mandarin, neroli, orange, palmarosa, rose maroc, rose otto, sandalwood, vetiver, ylang-ylang

Contra-indications:	**Purchasing Guide:**
None known	**Price Range:** medium

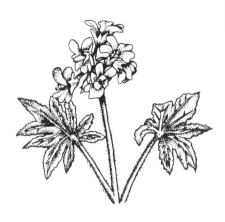

Geranium

(Pelargonium graveolens) Botanical Family: Geraniaceae

Plant growing up to 1 metre high, with pink-white flowers.
Plant Part used: leaves and flowering tops
Method of Extraction: steam distillation
Countries of Production: Egypt, Reunion (Bourbon geranium), China
Fragrance: flowery, green, rose-like
Note: middle
Main Chemical Components:
citronellol, geraniol, linalol, citronellyl formate
General Effect: relaxing, balancing

Indicated for:

The Face	The Body
acne	anxiety
ageing skin	balancing
broken capillaries	calming
circulation	circulation
combination	congestion
congested skin	depression
dry skin	fatigue
eczema	fluid retention
flaking skin	pre-menstrual tension
inflammation	relaxing
mature skin	revitalisation
normal skin	sluggishness
oily skin	stress
revitalisation	tension
skin irritations	toning
skin tone	varicose veins
sliggishness	

Body Blending Guide:
Bergamot, bois de rose, camomile roman, clary sage, cypress, fennel, frankincense, ginger, grapefruit, jasmine, juniper, lavender, lemon, mandarin, neroli, orange, palma rosa, peppermint, petitgrain, rose maroc, rosemary, rose otto, sandalwood, violet leaf, ylang-ylang

Contra-indications:
None known

Purchasing Guide:
Price Range: low

Ginger	
(Zingiber officinale) Botanical Family: *Zingiberacae*	

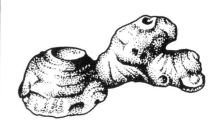

Perennial herb over 1 metre high, with yellow and purple flowers, long thin leaves and the rhizome growing underground.
Plant Part used: fresh or dried rhizome
Method of Extraction: steam distillation
Countries of Production: India, China, West Indies
Fragrance: characteristic of ginger
Note: middle to base
Main Chemical Components:
α, β-zingiberene, geranial, ar-curcumene, 1,8-cineole, neral
General Effect: stimulating, warming

Indicated for:

The Face	The Body
Not used in facial treatments	aches and pains chilliness circulation stimulating digestive problems fatigue sluggishness stiffness stimulating

Body Blending Guide:
Bergamot, cedarwood, frankincense, geranium, jasmine, mandarin, marjoram, orange, palmarosa, patchouli, petitgrain, rose maroc, sandalwood, ylang-ylang

Contra-indications:	**Purchasing Guide:**
Can cause irritation – use with care. Avoid using in water-immersion methods.	**Price Range:** medium

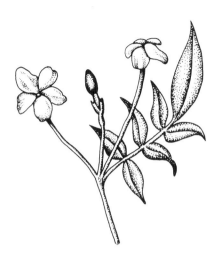

Jasmine (Absolute)

(Jasmininum grandiflorum, J. officinale) Botanical Family: *Oleaceae*

A climbing bush that grows up to 10 metres high, with dark green leaves and small, white star-shaped flowers.

Plant Part used: flowers
Method of Extraction: enfleurage; solvent or CO_2 extraction
Countries of Production: France, India, Egypt
Fragrance: deep, sweet, exotic floral
Note: middle
Main Chemical Components:
benzyl acetate, linalol, geraniol, benzyl benzoate, cis-jasmone, indole
General Effect: relaxing, balancing

Indicated for:

The Face	The Body
ageing skin	anxiety
dry skin	calming
mature skin	depression
normal skin	relaxing
revitalisation	scarring
scarring	skin revitalisation
	stress
	tension
	toning

Body Blending Guide:
Bergamot, geranium, ginger, lemon, mandarin, neroli, orange, palma rosa, patchouli, petitgrain, rose maroc, rose otto, sandalwood, violet leaf, ylang-ylang

Contra-indications:	**Purchasing Guide:**
None known	**Price Range:** high

Juniper Berry

(Juniperus communis) Botanical Family: Cupressaceae

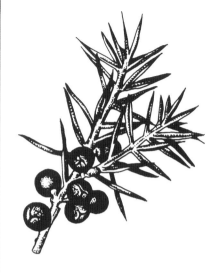

A large shrub with needle-like leaves. Only the female variety produce the bluish grey berries.

Plant Part used: berries
Method of Extraction: steam distillation
Countries of Production: Hungary, Bulgaria, Russia, Croatia
Fragrance: fresh, fruity, woody
Note: top
Main Chemical Components:
α-pinene, sabinene, myrcene, terpineol-4-ol, p-cymene
General Effect: energising, refreshing

Indicated for:

The Face	The Body
acne	cellulite
congested skin	congestion
eczema	detoxification
inflamed skin	eczema
irritated skin	fluid retention
itching	inflammation
oily skin	psoriasis
psoriasis	rashes
puffy skin	sluggishness
rashes	swelling
sluggishness	

Body Blending Guide:
Bergamot, cedarwood, clary sage, cypress, eucalyptus, fennel, frankincense, geranium, grapefruit, lavender, lemon, lemongrass, mandarin, pine, rosemary, vetiver, violet leaf

Contra-indications
To be avoided during pregnancy and lactation.
Can cause irritation on sensitive skins – use with care.
To be avoided by those with kidney problems.

Purchasing Guide:
Price Range: medium

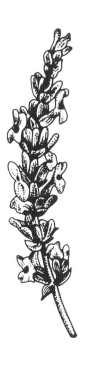

Lavender

(Lavendula angustifolia, L. officinalis) Botanical Family: *Lamiaceae* (or *Labiate*)

A herbaceous plant growing over a metre high, producing long, stick-like woody stems, with purple or violet flowers resembling tightly-packed pods.

Plant Part used: flowering tops
Method of Extraction: steam distillation
Countries of Production: France, Bulgaria, China, England, Tasmania, Croatia
Fragrance: fresh, light, floral
Note: top
Main Chemical Components: linalyl acetate, linalol, lavandulyl, caryophyllene, 1,8-cineol, 3-octanone
General Effect: relaxing, calming

Indicated for:

The Face	The Body
blemished	aches and pains
burns (use undiluted only)	acne
combination skin	anxiety
delicate skin	balancing
dry skin	burns (use undiluted only)
eczema	calming
infections	eczema
inflammation	exhaustion
itching	inflammation
normal skin	insomnia
oily skin	itching
psoriasis	nervous conditions
rashes	pre-menstrual tension
scarring	psoriasis rashes relaxing
seborrhoea	scarring
sensitive skin	skin infections
sun burn	spasms
sun damage	stress
	tension

Body Blending Guide:
Bergamot, black pepper, bois de rose, camomile german, camomile roman, cedarwood, clary sage, cypress, eucalyptus, geranium, jasmine, juniper, lemongrass, mandarin, marjoram, palmarosa, patchouli, peppermint, rose maroc, rosemary, rose otto, tea tree, thyme linalol, violet leaf

Contra-indications:	**Purchasing Guide:**
None known	**Price Range:** moderate

Lemon

(Citrus limonum) Botanical Family: Rutaceae

A small tree with white flowers and yellow citrus fruits.
Plant Part used: fresh fruit peel
Method of Extraction: cold expression
Countries of Production: Italy/Sicily, USA, Argentina, Spain, Israel
Fragrance: characteristic of lemon
Note: top
Main Chemical Components:
limonene, β-pinene, γ-terpinene, myrcene, α-pinene
General Effect: energising, refreshing

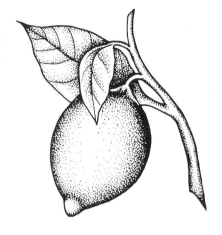

Indicated for:

The Face	The Body
acne	cleansing
blemishes	congestion
cleansing	depression
combination skin	eczema
congested skin	exhaustion
dilated pores	fatigue
infections	revitalising
normal skin	sluggishness
oily skin	soothing
puffiness	tension
purifying	
revitalisation	
sluggishness	
toning	

Blending Guide:
Basil, black pepper, geranium, jasmine, lavender, marjoram, palma rosa, petitgrain, rose maroc, rosemary, rose otto, tea tree, vetiver, violet leaf, ylang-ylang

Contra-indications:
Should not be used prior to sunbed use, or before going in prolonged sunlight.
Avoid using in water-immersion methods unless diluted.

Purchasing Guide:
Shelf-life of only about 9 months
Price Range: low

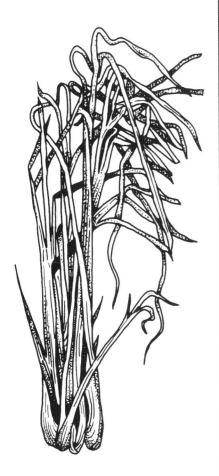

Lemongrass

(Cymbopogon flexuosus) Botanical Family: *Graminacea*

Perennial grass growing over a metre high. The long narrow leaves bend, and fold towards the ground.
Plant Part used: leaves
Method of Extraction: steam distillation
Countries of Production: India, Sri Lanka, Guatamala
Fragrance: lemony, hay-like
Note: middle
Main Chemical Components:
citral, limonene
General Effect: invigorating, strengthening

Indicated for:

The Face	The Body
acne	cellulite
blemishes	congestion
dilated pores	exhaustion
infections	sluggishness
oily skin	stiffness
seborrhoea	stimulating
	toning

Body Blending Guide:
Basil, bergamot, black pepper, cedarwood, clary sage, cypress, fennel, geranium, ginger, lavender, lemon, marjoram, orange, palmarosa, patchouli, petitgrain, rosemary, tea tree, vetiver, ylang-ylang

Contra-indications:
Can cause skin irritation – use with care, especially on the face

Purchasing Guide:
Price Range: low

Mandarin

(Citrus reticulata) Botanical Family: *Rutaceae*

A small evergreen tree, producing fragrant, cream-coloured flowers and small, loose skinned fruits, orange in colour.
Plant Part used: fruit rind
Method of Extraction: cold expression
Countries of Production: USA, Brazil, Algeria, Tunisia, Argentina
Fragrance: sweet, fruity, citrus
Note: top
Main Chemical Components:
limonene, γ-terpinolene, α-pinene, β-pinene
General Effect: calming, refreshing

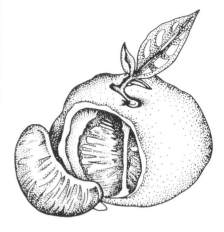

Indicated for:

The Face	The Body
combination skin	anxiety
oily skin	balancing
scarring	calming
	convalescence
	fatigue
	general body oil
	relaxing
	stretch marks
	tension

Body Blending Guide:
Black pepper, camomile roman, clary sage, frankincense, geranium, grapefruit, jasmine, juniper, lemon, neroli, palmarosa, patchouli, petitgrain, rose maroc, rose otto, sandalwood, ylang-ylang

Contra-indications:
Should not be used prior to sunbed use, or before going in prolonged sunlight

Purchasing Guide:
Price Range: low

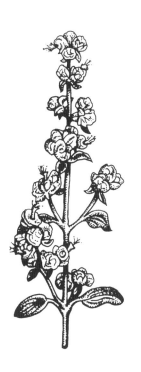

Marjoram (Sweet)	
(Origanum Marjorana) Botanical Family: *Labiatiae*	

Bushy herb with dark green leaves and small white flowers
Plant Part used: flowering herb
Method of Extraction: steam distillation
Countries of Production: France, Tunisia, Egypt
Fragrance: soft, characteristic of the herb
Note: middle
Main Chemical Components:
terpinen-4-ol, γ-terpineol, linalyl acetate, cis-sabinene hydrate, p-cymene, linalol
General Effect: calming, strengthening

Indicated for:

The Face	The Body
Not to be used in facial treatments	aches and pains congestion exhaustion fortifying muscular spasm stiffness strengthening stress tension warming

Blending Guide:
Basil, bergamot, black pepper, clary sage, juniper, lavender, lemon, orange, rosemary, thyme linalol

Contra-indications: None known	**Purchasing Guide:** **Price Range:** low

Melissa

(Melissa officinalis) Botanical Family: Labiatae (or Lamiaceae)

A bushy herb growing to 1 metre, with small, lemon-scented, serrated leaves. The pink-white flowers grow near the ground.
Plant Part used: flowering tops, leaves and stems
Method of Extraction: steam distillation of fresh material
Countries of Production: France, Ireland, Hungary, Italy
Fragrance: light, green, citrus
Note: middle
Main Chemical Components:
geraniol, neral, caryophyllene, germacrene, 1-octen-3-ol, citronellal
General Effect: uplifting, soothing

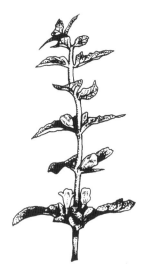

Indicated for:

The Face	The Body
acne	acne
herpes simplex	depression
infections	herpes simplex
oily skin	nervous tension
purifying	purifying
revitalising	revitalising
	skin infections
	stress

Body Blending Guide: *Use small quantities*
Camomile roman, frankincense, geranium, jasmine, neroli, petitgrain, rose maroc, rose otto, violet leaf

Contra-indications:	**Purchasing Guide:**
May cause skin irritation – use with care.	**Price Range:** high
Ensure only absolutely pure melissa is used, and not a reconstituted substitute.	

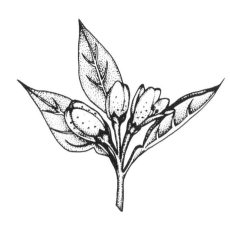

Neroli

(Citrus aurantium, C. brigaradia, C. vulgaris) Botanical Family: *Rutacea*

The bitter-orange tree, standing up to 10 metres high, produces the small, white, waxy flowers from which this oil is made.

Plant Part used: flowers
Method of Extraction: steam distillation
Countries of Production: Tunisia, Algeria, France, Italy
Fragrance: highly radiant, sweet, floral
Note: top to middle
Main Chemical Components:
linalyl acetate, linalol, geraniol, nerolidol, neroli
General Effect: balancing, soothing

Indicated for:

The Face	The Body
acne	anxiety
ageing	calming
broken capillaries	exhaustion
dry skin	insomnia
eczema	light muscular spasm
inflamed skin	nervous tension
mature skin	relaxing
revitalisation	scarring
sensitive skin	skin revitalisation
skin elasticity	stress
toning	tension

Body Blending Guide:
Bergamot, bois de rose, camomile roman, geranium, jasmine, lavender, lemon, mandarin, orange, petitgrain, rose maroc, rose otto, sandalwood, ylang-ylang

Contra-indications:
None known

Purchasing Guide:
Sometimes called 'orange blossom' – especially in hydrolat form
Price Range: high

Orange

(Citrus aurantium, C. sinensis, C. brigarde) Botanical Family: *Rutacea*

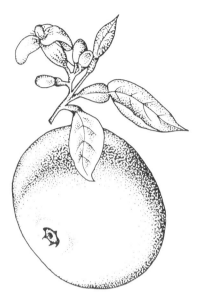

Small tree with dark leaves, white flowers and bright orange round fruits.

Plant Part used: peel
Method of Extraction: cold-pressed
Countries of Production: Brazil, Israel, Morocco, Tunisia, Algeria, USA
Fragrance: characteristic of orange
Note: top
Main Chemical Components:
limonene, myrecene, sabinene, α-pinene
General Effect: energising, strengthening

Indicated for:

The Face	The Body
blemishes	balancing
cleansing	depression
combination skin	digestive problems
congested skin	exhaustion
dilated pores	general body oil
oily skin	sluggishness
puffiness	swelling
	tension
	toning
	uplifting

Body Blending Guide:
Bergamot, black pepper, frankincense, geranium, ginger, jasmine, juniper, lemon, marjoram, neroli, patchouli, petitgrain, rose maroc, rose otto, sandalwood, vetiver, violet leaf, ylang-ylang

Contra-indications:
Should not be used prior to sunbed use, or before going in prolonged sunlight

Purchasing Guide:
Citrus aurantium is the source of 'bitter orange' essential oil, while 'sweet orange' is expressed from Citrus sinensis
Price Range: low

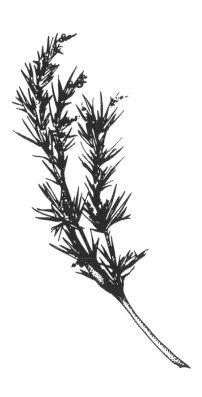

Palmarosa

(Cymbopogon martini Stapf.) Botanical Family: *Graminaceae*

A grass with long stems that end in tufts, and small yellow flowers. The grass is harvested before flowering, and is distilled either fresh or dried.

Plant Part used: grass
Method of Extraction: steam distillation
Countries of Production: India, Madagascar, Nepal
Fragrance: lemony, floral, with hint of rose
Note: middle
Main Chemical Components:
geraniol, granyl acetate, linalol, β-caryophyllene
General Effect: refreshing, stimulating

Indicated for:

The Face	The Body
acne	body blemishes
ageing	congestion
balancing	detoxifying
cleansing	digestive problems
eczema	exhaustion
fungal infection	fluid retention
infections	relaxing
mature skin	skin infections
oily skin	swellings
regenerative	
seborrhoea	

Body Blending Guide:
Bergamot, clary sage, frankincense, geranium, ginger, juniper, lemon, lemongrass, mandarin, orange, patchouli, petitgrain, rose maroc, rosemary, rose otto, sandalwood, ylang-ylang

Contra-indications:
None known

Purchasing Guide:
Price Range: low

Patchouli

(Pogostemon Cablin) Botanical Family: Labiatae

Herbaceous, perennial bush growing a metre high. Hairy leaves, white flowers with purple hue.
Plant Part used: non-flower leaves
Method of Extraction: Steam distillation of sun-dried, slightly fermented leaves
Countries of Production: Indonesia, India
Fragrance: sweet, earthy
Note: base
Main Chemical Components:
patchouli alcohol, α-bulnescene, α-guaiene, seychellene α-patchouline
General Effect: relaxing

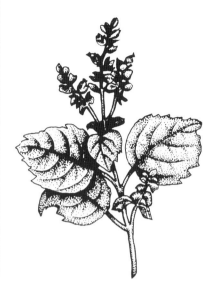

Indicated for:

The Face	The Body
acne	anxiety
blemishes	cellulite
combination skin	depression
normal skin	fluid retention
oily skin	inflammation
puffiness	pre-menstrual tension
seborrhoea	rashes
toning	skin blemishes
	stress
	swelling
	toning

Body Blending Guide:
Bergamot, black pepper, camomile german, cedarwood, clary sage, frankincense, geranium, ginger, jasmine, lemongrass, mandarin, neroli, orange, rose maroc, sandalwood, vetiver, ylang-ylang

Contra-indications:	**Purchasing Guide:**
None known	**Price Range:** medium

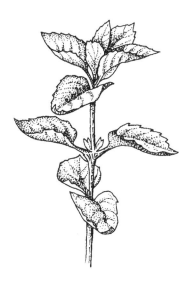

Peppermint

(Mentha piperita) Botanical Family: Lamiaceae (Labiatae)

Perennial plant half a metre high, with small leaves and pink-mauve flowers.
Plant Part used: all plant above ground
Method of Extraction: steam distillation
Countries of Production: USA, Russia, China, Tasmania
Fragrance: characteristic of peppermint
Note: middle-to-top
Main Chemical Components:
menthol, menthone, 1,8-cineole, methyl acetate, menthofuran
General Effect: stimulating, invigorating

Indicated for:

The Face	The Body
Use in extremely low amounts, keeping well away from the eyes	bloating
combination skin	bodily congestion
oily skin	cramp
purifying	digestive problems
sinus congestion	dysmenorrhoea
	fatigue
	inflammation
	muscular spasms
	nervous tension
	sluggishness
	stiffness
	stimulating

Body Blending Guide:
Basil, black pepper, cypress, eucalyptus, geranium, grapefruit, juniper, lavender, lemon, pine, rosemary, tea tree

Contra-indications:
Can cause skin irritation – use with care.
Avoid using in water-immersion methods.
To be avoided during pregnancy and lactation.

Purchasing Guide:
Price Range: low

Petitgrain

(Citrus aurantium, ss C. amara, C. brigaradier) Botanical Family: *Rutacea*

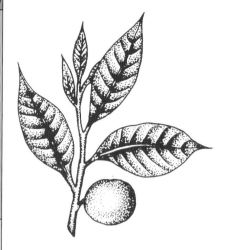

The orange tree. Petitgrain oil is distilled from the dark, glossy leaves, the smallest twigs and the fruit buds that remain after the flowers have fallen. In high-quality oil, the tiny, green, unripe fruits are also included.

Plant Part used: leaves, twigs, buds (and possibly the unripe fruit)

Method of Extraction: steam distillation

Countries of Production: Paraguay, France, Italy, Algeria, Tunisia, Morocco

Fragrance: a green, woody, floral

Note: middle

Main Chemical Components:
linalyl acetate, linalol, terpineol, myrcene, geraniol

General Effect: refreshing, balancing

Indicated for:

The Face	The Body
acne	anxiety
ageing skin	balancing
blemishes	depression
cleansing	exhaustion
mature skin	general body oil
oily skin	insomnia
puffiness	muscular spasm
toning effect	nervous tension
	relaxing
	stress conditions
	tension

Body Blending Guide:
Basil, bergamot, cedarwood, clary sage, cypress, frankincense, geranium, jasmine, lavender, lemon, mandarin, marjoram, neroli, orange, palmarosa, patchouli, rose maroc, rosemary, rose otto, sandalwood, ylang-ylang

Contra-indications:	**Purchasing Guide:**
None known	**Price Range:** low

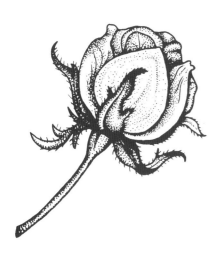

Rose Maroc (Absolute)	67
(Rosa centifolia) Botanical Family: *Rosaceae*	

Rose bush growing up to 2 metres high, sometimes trained to grow vertically, when it produces hundreds of blossoms.
Plant Part used: flesh flower heads
Method of Extraction: enfleurage; solvent extraction
Countries of Production: Morocco, Turkey, Egypt, France
Fragrance: deep, soft, hypnotic rose
Note: middle to base
Main Chemical Components:
ethanol, citronellol, geraniol, nerol, stearopten
General Effect: relaxing, calming

Indicated for:

The Face	The Body
ageing skin	calming
dull skin	circulation stimulating
mature skin	depression
normal skin	dysmenorrhoea
revitalising	harmonising
toning	infertility
	insomnia
	menopause
	pre-menstrual tension
	relaxing
	revitalising

Body Blending Guide:
Frankincense, geranium, jasmine, lemon, mandarin, neroli, palmarosa, sandalwood, ylang-ylang

Contra-indications:	**Purchasing Guide:**
None known	**Price Range:** high

Rose Otto (Rose Bulgar)

(Rosa damascena) Botanical Family: *Rosaceae*

Annually flowering rose bush, growing to over 1 metre. Only the pink variety is used.

Plant Part used: fresh flowers
Method of Extraction: steam distillation
Countries of Production: Bulgaria, Turkey, France
Fragrance: fresh, rose floral
Note: middle
Main Chemical Components:
citronellol, geraniol, nerol, stearopten, farnesol, phenyl ethanol
General Effect: soothing, calming

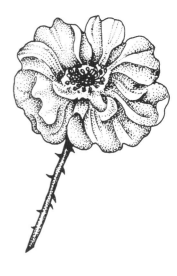

Indicated for:

The Face	The Body
ageing skin	anxiety
broken capillaries	bloating
dry skin	calming
flaking skin	circulation stimulating
normal skin	coldness
nourishing	depression
oily skin	dysmenorrhea
regenerating	infertility
revitalising	menopausal
scarring	pre-menstrual tension
sensitive skin	relaxing
swollen tissues	scarring
	spasms
	stress

Body Blending Guide:
Camomile roman, geranium, jasmine, lavender, lemon, neroli, petitgrain, sandalwood

Contra-indications:	**Purchasing Guide:**
None known	**Price Range:** high

Rosemary

(Rosmarinus officinalis) Botanical Family: *Labiatae (Labiaceae)*

A spiked-leaf bush growing to over 1 metre. The stem is gnarled and twisted, with long, thin branches. Tiny blue flowers grow among the spiked leaves.

Plant Part used: leaves and twigs – flowering tops
Method of Extraction: steam distillation
Countries of Production: Tunisia, France, Spain, Morocco
Fragrance: characteristic of the herb
Note: middle to top
Main Chemical Components:
1,8-cineole, α-pinene, camphor, camphene, β-pinene, bornyl acetate
General Effect: stimulating, invigorating

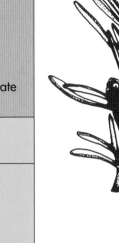

Indicated for:

The Face	The Body
acne	aches and pains
balancing	breathing conditions
circulation stimulating	cellulite
combination skin	circulation stimulating
congested skin	congestion
detoxifying	fatigue
dull skin	fluid retention
oily skin	fortifying
seborrhoea	muscle toning
sinus congestion	sluggishness
	stiffness
	stimulating

Body Blending Guide:
Basil, bergamot, black pepper, cedarwood, clary sage, cypress, eucalyptus, frankincense, geranium, grapefruit, juniper, lavender, lemon, mandarin, marjoram, palma rosa, peppermint, tea tree, thyme linalol

Contra-indications:
Can cause skin irritation – use with care.
To be avoided during pregnancy and lactation.
To be avoided by those with epilepsy.

Purchasing Guide:
Price Range: low

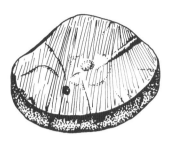

Sandalwood

(Santalum album) Botanical Family: Santalaceae

An evergreen tree growing over 20 metres, with orange flowers, taking nutrients from the roots of nearby trees.
Plant Part used: chipped wood
Method of Extraction: steam distillation
Countries of Production: India, Indonesia
Fragrance: sweet, balsamic, woody
Note: base
Main Chemical Components:
α-santalol, β-santalol, α-santalene, β-santalene
General Effect: relaxing, strengthening

Indicated for:

The Face	The Body
ageing	anxiety
cracked and chapped	balancing
dehydrated	bloating
dry skin	calming
flaking skin	depression
infections	exhaustion
irritated skin	fortifying
itching	inflammation
mature	nervousness
normal skin	relaxing
redness	stress
seborrhoea	tension
sensitive skin	
soothing	
toning	

Body Blending Guide:
Black pepper, camomile roman, geranium, jasmine, lavender, lemon, mandarin, neroli, orange, palmarosa, petitgrain, rose maroc, rose otto, ylang-ylang

Contra-indications:	**Purchasing Guide:**
None known	**Price Range:** medium

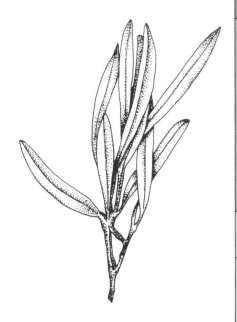

Tea Tree

(Melaleuca alternifolia) Botanical Family: *Myrtaceae*

A tree that is cut to bush-size when under cultivation, to around 1½ metres. The slim leaves are around 8 cm long.

Plant Part used: leaves and twigs
Method of Extraction: steam distillation
Country of Production: Australia
Fragrance: sharp, medicinal, camphorous
Note: middle
Main Chemical Components:
terpinen-4-ol, γ-terpinene, α-terpinene, 1,8-cineole, α-terpineol, p-cymene
General Effect: stimulating, refreshing

Indicated for:

The Face	The Body
acne	bacterial infection
bacterial infection	fungal infections
blemishes	rashes
itching	soreness
psoriasis	
purifying	
rashes	
seborrhoea	
sinus congestion	

Body Blending Guide:
Basil, bergamot, camomile german, cypress, eucalyptus radiata, juniper, lavender, lemon, marjoram, peppermint, thyme linalol

Contra-indications:
None known

Purchasing Guide:
Price Range: low

Thyme Linalol

(Thymus vulgaris – chemotype linalol) Botanical Family: *Labiatae*

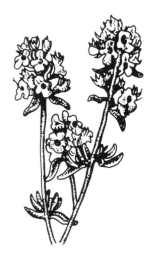

Perennial dwarf shrub growing to 20 cm high, with woody stems, tiny leaves and pink-lilac flowers.
Plant Part used: flowering tops
Method of Extraction: steam distillation
Countries of Production: France, Spain
Fragrance: soft, woody, herby
Note: middle
Main Chemical Components:
linalol, β-carophyllene, thymol, p-cymene
General Effect: stimulating, soothing

Indicated for:

The Face	The Body
acne	blemishes
blemishes	cellulite
congested skin	congestion
congestion	fungal infections
detoxification	general infections
skin impurities	muscular spasm
skin infections	muscular tension
viral infections	stiffness
	stimulating
	sluggishness
	viral infections

Body Blending Guide:
Cedarwood, geranium, grapefruit, lemon, marjoram, palmarosa, rosemary, tea tree

Contra-indications:
Can cause skin irritation – use with care
Avoid using in water-immersion methods unless diluted.
To be avoided during pregnancy and lactation.

Purchasing Guide:
This profile relates to Thyme Linalol only. No other thymes are recommended for beauty purposes.
Price Range: medium

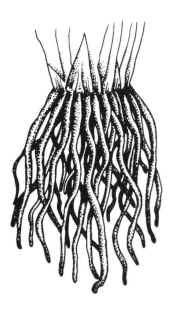

Vetiver

(Vetiveria zizanoides) Botanical Family: *Gramineae (Graminaceae)*

Perennial grass growing up to 2 metres high. The roots are very long and rhizomatous.
Plant Part used: washed, dried, sliced, or ground, roots
Method of Extraction: steam distillation
Countries of Production: Indonesia, India, Haiti
Fragrance: earthy, musty
Note: base
Main Chemical Components:
benzoic acid, furfural, vetiverol, α-vetivone, β-vetivone
General Effect: relaxing

Indicated for:

The Face	The Body
acne	anxiety
ageing skin	balancing
blemished skin	exhaustion
dull skin	insomnia
mature skin	menopause
oily skin	stress
toning	tension

Body Blending Guide:
Bergamot, geranium, lavender, lemon, lemongrass, mandarin, orange, sandalwood

Contra-indications:
None known

Purchasing Guide:
Should be a soft aroma, not harsh
Price Range: low

Violet Leaf (Absolute)

(Viola odorata) Botanical Family: Violaceae

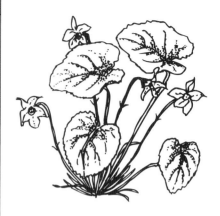

Small plant with dark, heart shaped green leaves and small violet flowers.

Plant Part used: leaves
Method of Extraction: distillation; solvent extraction
Countries of Production: France
Fragrance: reminiscent of green undergrowth
Note: base
Main Chemical Components:
2-trans-6-cis-nonadien-1-al, n-hexanol, n-octen-2-ol-1, benzyl alcohol, tertiary octenol, hexenol
General Effect: calming

Indicated for:

The Face	The Body
acne	anxiety
ageing skin	congested tissues
detoxifying	detoxifying
dilated pores	tension
dull skin	tissue and skin tone
elasticity of tissues	
mature skin	
muscle tone	
puffiness	
tired complexion	

Body Blending Guide:
Bergamot, bois de rose, geranium, lavender, neroli, orange, palmarosa, rose maroc

Contra-indications: None known	**Purchasing Guide:** **Price Range:** High

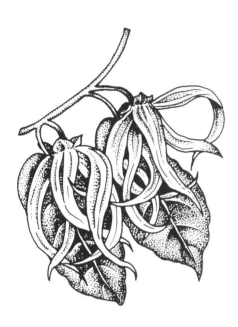

Ylang-Ylang (Extra)

(Canangium odorata forma genuina) Botanical Family: *Anonaceae*

A 7-metre high tree that produces large, highly scented, drooping, flowers.
Plant Part used: flowers
Method of Extraction: steam distillation
Countries of Production: Madagascar (Comoros Islands)
Fragrance: intense, exotic floral
Note: middle
Main Chemical Components:
benzyl acetate, p-carsyl methylether, linalol, methyl benzoate, sesquiterpenes
General Effect: calming

Indicated for:

The Face	The Body
balancing	anxiety
combination	balancing
oily	insomnia
revitalisation	nervous conditions
scarring	pre-menstrual tension
soothing	relaxing
toning	spasm
	stress
	tension
	tissue revitalising
	toning

Body Blending Guide:
Bergamot, geranium, ginger, grapefruit, jasmine, lemon, mandarin, neroli, orange, palmarosa, patchouli, petitgrain, rose maroc, sandalwood

Contra-indications:
None known

Purchasing Guide:
There are four grades, and the chemistry is very different between them. Only use 'extra quality' for therapeutic work.

Price Range: medium

The Salon and Retail Sales Potential

Within the beauty salon, essential oils can be used in many different ways:

- In treatment rooms or cubicles, they are incorporated into individual, tailor-made facials and body treatments, used in nail and after-care treatments, and hair-removal after-care products.
- They can be used in hydrotherapy and any water-based treatment.
- In a diffuser, they can impart a pleasant fragrance in wash-room areas.
- In a diffuser, they can be used to impart a relaxing atmosphere to the reception area.
- Essential oils and products containing essential oils can be sold retail in the reception area.

USING ESSENTIAL OIL IN THE TREATMENT ROOM OR CUBICLE

Ventilation

Different essential oils may be used in facial and body treatments on various clients during the course of the day, and these different aromas might be incompatible with each other. For example, a stimulating aroma might be appropriate for the first client, and a relaxing aroma for the second client. If the stimulating aroma used in the first treatment is still permeating the room during the second treatment, it may negate the relaxing effect of the aroma then being used. It is important, therefore, to refresh the air in the treatment room by taking one or more of the following steps:

- open the window between treatments;
- increase the power of the air-conditioning system for several minutes between treatments;
- open the door of the cubicle between treatments.

TIP

Have an aromatherapy product reference book available in the reception area. This can be referred to if staff do not know the answer to questions asked by clients regarding the properties of essential oils.

TIP

When a bottle of essential oil is to be used within the salon, write the date on the label when it is taken into stock. Essential oils keep their therapeutic value for, on average, two years. After this time, an essential oil should not be used for therapeutic purposes, but it can be used as a fragrance in diffusers around the salon.

HEALTH AND SAFETY

Adequate ventilation is important for the health and safety of the therapist who may be inhaling essential oils all day during the course of her work.

To help prevent an accumulation of essential oils in her body, the beauty therapist should drink plain water during the course of the day to help flush the system out, and get plenty of fresh air between treatments.

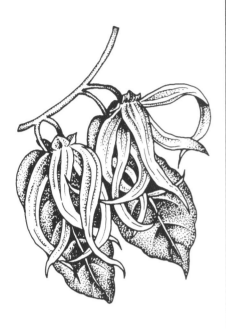

Ylang-Ylang (Extra)

(Canangium odorata forma genuina) Botanical Family: *Anonaceae*

A 7-metre high tree that produces large, highly scented, drooping, flowers.
Plant Part used: flowers
Method of Extraction: steam distillation
Countries of Production: Madagascar (Comoros Islands)
Fragrance: intense, exotic floral
Note: middle
Main Chemical Components:
benzyl acetate, p-carsyl methylether, linalol, methyl benzoate, sesquiterpenes
General Effect: calming

Indicated for:

The Face	The Body
balancing	anxiety
combination	balancing
oily	insomnia
revitalisation	nervous conditions
scarring	pre-menstrual tension
soothing	relaxing
toning	spasm
	stress
	tension
	tissue revitalising
	toning

Body Blending Guide:
Bergamot, geranium, ginger, grapefruit, jasmine, lemon, mandarin, neroli, orange, palmarosa, patchouli, petitgrain, rose maroc, sandalwood

Contra-indications:
None known

Purchasing Guide:
There are four grades, and the chemistry is very different between them. Only use 'extra quality' for therapeutic work.

Price Range: medium

Professional Blending Techniques

The way in which essential oils are blended will very much depend on the intended use of the finished product. As a general rule, products intended for the face will have a lower percentage of essential oil, while products intended for use on the body will have a higher percentage of essential oil. The essential oils and the base oils chosen, along with their relative proportions, will depend upon the physical condition of each individual client.

Blending for beauty purposes is often more effective when the ingredients have had time to amalgamate and mature together. For this reason, pre-preparing blends is an important aspect of this subject.

The advice in this chapter should be viewed as an introduction to the subject of blending. Those trained in clinical or medical aromatherapy will use additional blending techniques, and will have acquired the skills to prepare individual products that can be used immediately on the client. Custom blending for aesthetic aromatherapy is a specialised subject that requires extensive study which provides the therapist with more options and flexibility.

There are three basic techniques that the beauty therapist using aromatherapy should become familiar with: *Pre-prepared blends, Immediate individual client blends and Home-use blends*. Each of these is discussed later in this chapter.

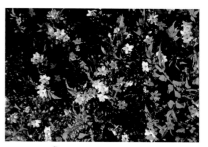
Jasmine flowers

EQUIPMENT REQUIRED

The best equipment to use when blending essential oils or base oils and other carrier mediums is glass, as it is easily sterilised, inactive and non-porous. You will need:

- **essential oils;**
- **carrier oils and other carrier mediums;**
- **glass measuring cylinders in various measuring volumes**
  to accurately measure amounts of essential oil;
- **glass measuring jugs**
  to measure base oils or other carrier mediums;

TIP

Plastics and ceramics should never be used to store or blend essential oils. See Storage in Chapter 6.

BOTTLES AND CONTAINERS

Amber bottles and containers can be purchased from many beauty supply companies, specialist aromatherapy essential oil suppliers and, sometimes, your local pharmacy. They come in varying sizes. A facial only requires a very small amount of oil, so in general the beauty therapist needs to purchase the smallest bottles available. For facials only, it is quite helpful to have on hand very small glass bowls, from which the oil can easily be taken during treatment.

These small glass bowls are available from laboratory supply companies and professional catering suppliers.

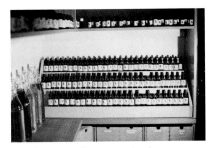

A selection of essential oils and (at left) base oils

- **glass funnels**
  for ease of bottling;
- **glass stirring rods**
  to thoroughly stir and agitate the blends;
- **amber glass bottles**
  in varying sizes to use during treatments and for storage;
- **small glass dishes**
  for use during treatments;
- **glass droppers**
  to accurately measure drops of essential oil;
- **scales**
  accurate enough to measure minute amounts of essential oils and other substances (if available);
- **blending sheets;**
- **labels.**

(1) PRE-PREPARED BLENDS

There are a number of common skin types, and essential oil blends or products can be pre-prepared for clients with these specific skin types. Although the beauty therapist *preparing* these blends requires specialist knowledge of essential oil synergy and aroma-chemistry, the beauty therapist *using* these products on a client does not. It is essential, however, that the beauty therapist using these pre-prepared blends makes an accurate diagnosis of the client's skin type and beauty needs, and understands the therapeutic qualities of all the available prepared blends, so that a good match of client-to-product can be made.

This method is preferred in many beauty salons because of the speed and ease-of-use of these aromatherapy products.

Technique

Choosing the Appropriate Essential Oils

- First, determine the use to which the blend/product is to be put.
- Use the individual essential oil profiles in Chapter 4 to choose the appropriate essential oils. Check all aspects of the oil. Note any contra-indications of the essential oil(s).
- Make notes on the blending sheet.

Choosing the Correct Base Oil or Lotion

- After choosing the essential oils, it is equally important to carefully choose an appropriate base or carrier oil, combination of oils or lotion in which to mix the essential oil or blend of oils.
- You can choose one, single, base oil or a combination of base oils. Alternatively, choose a natural base lotion, cream or other base material

- Finally, check that your chosen essential oils are compatible with your chosen carrier/base.
- Make notes on the blending sheet.

Blending the Essential Oils

- Arrange your chosen essential oils in order of therapeutic value. The first will usually contribute the largest percentage of essential oil to the blend. The second will contribute the next largest percentage, and so on. Which essential oil has priority will depend on the effect it has been chosen to achieve, and the knowledge that the essential oil is appropriate for that task.
- For salon purposes, the easiest way to start is by measuring out the largest amount first (whether this is in drops, millilitres or grams), followed by adding the second largest amount, and blending them together. Then add the next largest volume of essential oil, blend together again well, and so on until all essential oils are blended in.
- Leave the essential oil blend to stand in an air-tight bottle in a cool, dark place, for at least 24 hours.

Blending the Base Oil or Lotion

- First blend together any small additions to the base, for example red carrot extract and evening primrose. Do this even if the total number of drops required is very few.
- Then add the next largest addition, and the next largest, and so on.
- Finally, add the main component of your base or lotion.
- At each stage, blend thoroughly before proceeding to the next stage.
- Let your final base stand in an air-tight bottle or container in a cool, dark place, for at least 24 hours before using.

Mixing the Essential Oils with the Base Carrier Oil or Lotion

- Add the base oil or lotion to the essential oils.
- Do this in small, incremental steps, mixing as you go.
- This is easily achieved if you use a bottle. Start with the essential oil mix in the empty bottle; add approximately 25 per cent of your base; replace the lid; roll the bottle between your hands, or shake it; undo the lid, and add further base; mix again, and so on until all the base has been added.
- Label the final blend, detailing its intended use, ingredients, date of preparation and any batch number.
- Let your final blend stand in an air-tight bottle or container in a cool, dark place, for at least 48 hours before using. This is so that all the ingredients have time to thoroughly intermingle or amalgamate.

TIP

To prolong the therapeutic life of pre-prepared blends, store them in a very cool place when not in use. The therapeutic qualities of a well-stored blend will remain active for a maximum of four months.

TIP

BASE LOTIONS AND CREAMS
Some companies sell unperfumed lotions and creams which could be used as base products for essential oils and hydrolats. These should only include pure, natural ingredients, and care must be taken to ensure these bases are compatible with essential oils.

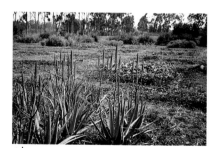

Aloe vera

DILUTION PERCENTAGES

Dilution of essential oil for the face See page 101–102	½ – 2%
Dilution of essential oil for the body See page 112	½ – 3%

Blending Sheets for Pre-Prepared Blends

For four very good reasons, it is very important to keep a record of all pre-prepared blends:

- If the individual blend is a success, it can be repeated exactly.
- Appropriate adjustments can be made to the original formulation, changing one or more essential oils, perhaps by just one or two drops. Accurate records allow changes to be monitored closely.
- If the individual blend is not proving effective, it can be altered with a full awareness of the changes being made.
- Contra-indications: if a blend causes a skin rash or other undesired effect, you can refer to the blending sheet to try to ascertain the cause. It could be that there is a problem with a particular essential oil, and you can see if the supplier or batch number is different from a previous successful blend which caused no contra-indications.

Pre-Prepared Blend for:	Side 1
	Write in the name of the product.
Company Name:	
Address, phone number etc.:	
Product:	* Part of the body the blend is required for. Skin type.
Product purpose:	* What it is to be used for – the aim it intends to achieve.
Prepared by:	* Name of the therapist responsible for preparing the blend.
To be used by:	* Names of therapists who can use the product.
Essential oils used, and volumes:	* The number of drops (millilitres or grams) of each essential oil. Can be expressed as a percentage of the carrier (below).
Carrier ingredients, and volumes:	* Base oils or other mediums used as the carrier. List all ingredients, and their volume.

Pre-Prepared Blend for:	**Side 2**

Reason for choosing these essential oils:	
Reason for choosing these base oils/other medium/ carrier:	
Name of essential oil supplier(s):	* Specify supplier of each oil.
Batch numbers:	* If known.
Use-by date:	* If known.
Testing:	* Details of any testing carried out on the effectiveness of the product.
Contra-indications:	* Any known problems that arise after the product has been used. Put date of any incident.
Date prepared: (1:) (2:) (3:) (4:) **Batch number:** (1:) (2:) (3:) (4:)	

(2) IMMEDIATE INDIVIDUAL CLIENT BLENDS

With immediate blending, a therapist makes a blend using essential oils and base oil(s) or another carrier medium, chosen specifically for a particular client, following the client consultation and observation. This is carried out 'on the spot' – in the cubicle or elsewhere within the salon.

This method should only be performed by those who have studied aromatherapy along with their beauty therapy training, or have been on an aromatherapy course for beauty therapists.

Technique

You will need a set of good, therapeutic-quality essential oils. Immediate blending should not be attempted with a kit of only, say, 12 essential oils, as this number is too limited to offer clients an individualised and effective treatment. For fragrance value, you will require essential oils from the top, middle and base note groups. And you will require several essential oils for all skin types groups, relevant to each of the following categories:

stimulating *energising* *relaxing*
stress relieving *skin toning* *analgesic*
skin cell *circulation* *anti-*
  proliferating *stimulating* *inflammatory*

Equipment Required

For immediate blending you will need:

- essential oils;
- good droppers (or essential oils supplied in bottles which have dropper inserts);
- clean, amber bottles, or a glass blending dish if preferred;
- glass measuring cup for base oils;
- glass stirring rod;
- small non-slip plastic mat;
- kitchen roll, or strong mop-up paper;
- an individual client blend sheet.

Immediate blending is carried after a full consultation and observation, often with the client present. The main difficulties arise when clients do not inform the therapist of what they consider minor factors or problems. For example, a client may say the problem is that their skin condition worsens pre-menstrually, but fail to tell you that they are on HRT (hormone replacement therapy), which can affect the skin condition. Another client may say they need stimulating because they are so tired, but fail to tell you they have insomnia due to stress – which is more likely the ultimate cause of the tiredness. A comprehensive consultation is the best insurance against misunderstandings or incomplete diagnosis, however choosing essential oils that have a general range of activity is also advisable.

Individual Client Blend Sheet and Therapist's Note-Sheet

Immediate blending for a specific client requires an individual blend sheet and, on the reverse, a therapist's note-sheet. When you are seeing many clients each day it is difficult to remember the individual requirements of the client, the treatment given on each occasion, and the changes made to treatment over time. Also, should another therapist need to take over a particular client's treatment, accurate records will allow them to follow through with appropriate treatment.

Client Blend Sheet	Side 1
Blending therapist:	* The name of the therapist blending the treatment.
Name:	* Name and address of client.
Address:	
Contact phone no.:	* Telephone number of client. Home, work/mobile.
Doctor's name and address:	* Name and address of the client's doctor.
Allergies:	* Any allergies to perfumes, skin care products, soaps, etc., foods such as wheat etc.
Medication:	* Any medication taken by the client, and for what reason.
Skin diagnosis/type:	* Skin type of the client.
Previous aromatherapy:	* Details of any previous aromatherapy treatments received.
Essential oil use:	* Has the client used essential oils before? If so, which?, and what brand(s)? Is the client using essential oils at present? For what purpose? Which oils?/brands?

Area treatment:	**Side 2** * What part of the body the blend/treatment is for. The problem, and the object of the treatment.
Essential oils:	* The essential oils chosen, and why.
Base/carrier:	* The base oil(s) or lotion chosen, and why.
Aromatherapy technique:	* The aromatherapy technique(s) being applied.
Home treatment:	* Any home treatment advice being given.
Product purchased:	* Details of any products purchased for client's use.
Notes:	* Write here any additional information offered by the client regarding their condition, along with any changes in the therapist's approach, or treatment. Other conditions found during treatment. Anything the therapist might have done differently, and will take into consideration on the next visit. Client's smell preferences.

Choosing the Appropriate Essential Oils

- Refer to the client consultation sheet for any existing medical condition(s), and make a note of any essential oils that cannot be used because of contra-indications.
- If the client is pregnant, also make a note of any essential oils that cannot be used because they are contra-indicated.
- Determine the client's skin type, and any skin conditions. Make a note on the *Client Blend Sheet*.
- Determine the use to which the blend/product is to be put. As well as the part of the body/face concerned, consider whether the blend should be relaxing, stimulating, energising, anti-stress or pain relieving. Make a note of your decision on the *Client Blend Sheet*.
- Also note the skin age – in this instance 'age' is not chronological, but biological – as some people's skin tone does not accurately reflect their chronological age.
- Choose the appropriate essential oils by referring to the individual essential oil profiles in Chapter 4. Take into consideration the listed psychological effects of the essential oils. Note any contra-indications of the essential oils chosen, and change your choice if appropriate.
- As far as possible, take a tip from perfumers and try to balance the blend with a base, middle and top note.
- When carrying out relaxation treatments, ask the client what type of aromas/perfumes she prefers – such as fruits, flowers, spices or the 'green' aroma of leaves. If appropriate for the treatment, try to use essential oils from the chosen category or categories.
- When carrying out specific skin treatments, whether to the face or body, it is not appropriate to let the client determine which essential oils are used. It is imperative that in these circumstances the essential oil chosen contains the correct properties for the treatment, as well as its aroma being acceptable to the client.
- A total of 3–5 essential oils will suffice for most client requirements, although a trained aromatherapist will use more, and more essential oils can be used as experience by the therapist is gained over time. The number of essential oils chosen will also depend on each salon's procedures, and on the individual therapist's training.
- Choose either a glass bottle, or a small glass dish, in which to blend your chosen essential oils.

> **HEALTH AND SAFETY**
> Medical conditions should not be treated professionally by beauty therapists. Any medical condition can only be treated by medical/clinical aromatherapists who are fully qualified and insured to do so.

Bottle Blending

Start by putting into the bottle the heaviest (by molecular weight) essential oil – the base note. Then put the middle note, then the top note (see *'Notes' – The Perfumer's Art* on page 28). Finally, to blend the essential oils well together, roll the bottle between your hands vigorously. It is at this stage that you add your chosen base oil(s) or lotion to the essential oils. Blend again by rolling the bottle vigorously between your hands, turning it upside a few times during this process, until the ingredients are thoroughly mixed.

Dish Blending

Measure out the correct volumes of essential oils directly into the dish, following the base, middle then top note procedure. Mix thoroughly with a glass stirring rod. Then add the correctly measured amount of base oil(s) or lotion to the dish, and stir thoroughly again.

It is important that the blend is very well mixed. As essential oils are often colourless, and therefore difficult to see when in a blend, they may gather in one area of the dish only – and be applied in greater amounts on one area of the face or body.

Because essential oils are volatile and evaporate quickly in both warm and cold conditions thereby losing their therapeutic value, blends prepared by this method should be used as quickly as possible.

(3) HOME-USE BLENDS

Often, after having an aesthetic aromatherapy treatment using essential oils, a client asks for a product they can use at home. If the blend used during treatment has been successful, a completely diluted version could be given to the client to take home. This would be made up of 50 per cent of the treatment blend, to which you add the same volume of additional base oil(s) or lotion.

You must bear in mind that you have no control over how a blend is used by other persons outside the salon environment, so care must be taken in the blending, in the essential oils used, and in the strength of the blend given for this purpose. By diluting the blend, you reduce the possibility of problems occurring.

- Before giving a client a home-use blend, you must first check with your insurance cover, or the salon's insurance policy, that it provides for product liability which includes preparing blends for clients to use at home.
- After giving a home-use blend to a client, make a note that you have done so on the *Client Blend Sheet*, as this is an addition to treatment.

Custom blending, whether for 'Immediate Individual Client Blends' or 'Home-Use Blends', is the province of the qualified aesthetic aromatherapist, who will have knowledge of aromatic chemistry and the cosmetic and medical application of essential oils.

HEALTH AND SAFETY
All persons preparing aesthetic aromatherapy treatments, whether using pre-prepared blends or preparing blends for immediate use on individual clients, should be insured for product liability as well as for professional liability.

The Salon and Retail Sales Potential

Within the beauty salon, essential oils can be used in many different ways:

- In treatment rooms or cubicles, they are incorporated into individual, tailor-made facials and body treatments, used in nail and after-care treatments, and hair-removal after-care products.
- They can be used in hydrotherapy and any water-based treatment.
- In a diffuser, they can impart a pleasant fragrance in wash-room areas.
- In a diffuser, they can be used to impart a relaxing atmosphere to the reception area.
- Essential oils and products containing essential oils can be sold retail in the reception area.

USING ESSENTIAL OIL IN THE TREATMENT ROOM OR CUBICLE

Ventilation

Different essential oils may be used in facial and body treatments on various clients during the course of the day, and these different aromas might be incompatible with each other. For example, a stimulating aroma might be appropriate for the first client, and a relaxing aroma for the second client. If the stimulating aroma used in the first treatment is still permeating the room during the second treatment, it may negate the relaxing effect of the aroma then being used. It is important, therefore, to refresh the air in the treatment room by taking one or more of the following steps:

- open the window between treatments;
- increase the power of the air-conditioning system for several minutes between treatments;
- open the door of the cubicle between treatments.

TIP

Have an aromatherapy product reference book available in the reception area. This can be referred to if staff do not know the answer to questions asked by clients regarding the properties of essential oils.

TIP

When a bottle of essential oil is to be used within the salon, write the date on the label when it is taken into stock. Essential oils keep their therapeutic value for, on average, two years. After this time, an essential oil should not be used for therapeutic purposes, but it can be used as a fragrance in diffusers around the salon.

HEALTH AND SAFETY

Adequate ventilation is important for the health and safety of the therapist who may be inhaling essential oils all day during the course of her work.

To help prevent an accumulation of essential oils in her body, the beauty therapist should drink plain water during the course of the day to help flush the system out, and get plenty of fresh air between treatments.

Do not diffuse essential oils in a treatment room or cubicle where any essential oil treatments will be carried out because:

- the essential oils used in the diffuser may conflict with the effect being sought during facial or body treatment;
- using essential oils in a diffuser can lead to aromatic overload for the therapist in the room;
- it is not necessary – the aromas being used in treatment will suffice in creating a pleasant atmosphere.

Face and Body Treatment Procedure

The most effective order in which to carry out a combined aromatherapy facial and body treatment is as follows:

- the back of the body;
- the front of the body;
- the face.
- The back is treated first so the essential oils applied to the back and around the vertebrae area – which have an effect upon the central nervous system – have time to be absorbed by the body.
- After working on an area of the back or front of the body, the area should be covered with either linens or towels, to prevent as far as possible the evaporation of the essential oils.
- Within a combined facial and body treatment, the facial will take up to fifteen minutes. This gives the essential oils, previously applied to the body, time to be absorbed. Also, while you are working on the facial area, the client's body will be able to rest and relax, taking full advantage of the treatment.

Why Face Last?

When clients lie face down or with their head turned sideways, the pressure on the couch-surface often creates creases or lines in the tissues of their face. This effect appears to be more pronounced when essential oils are used in facial treatments, during which lymphatic drainage techniques and reflex point pressure may have been applied. For these reasons, facial treatments are always performed last during aromatherapy facial and body treatments.

Equipment

When carrying out aromatherapy facial and body treatments, the following equipment should be available in the treatment room or cubicle:

- sterilised, pre-packaged eye cleaning solution; or eye-bath and distilled water;
- clean towels;
- means of washing/cleaning hands.

If carrying out individualised aromatherapy facial or body treatments, the following additional equipment is required:

- a range of essential oils;
- fresh, sterile glass equipment for each client;
- new amber bottles.

See page 76 in *Chapter Five – Professional Blending Techniques* for a complete list of the equipment required. The essential oils should be stored in a cool, dark place – away from any heat sources such as sunlight, radiators, warm-water pipes or light bulbs.

Hand Washing

During the course of a treatment, it may be necessary to wash or clean the hands. For example, if you use a strong essential oil treatment, that essential oil residue should not be on your hands when you continue treatment on another area of the face or body. Or, if you use an essential oil compress it will need to be squeezed out, and anything used in that compress will remain on your hands – so you will need to wash or wipe your hands before progressing to the next stage of treatment, which may very well involve another product.

If a sink and warm water are not available in the treatment room, ensure there are small wet towels to wipe your hands on between the various stages of treatment.

SALES POTENTIAL IN THE RECEPTION AREA

In the salon reception area, essential oils and aromatherapy products can be sold to:

- clients of aromatherapy treatments;
- other clients;
- visitors.

As with any salon product, good product knowledge is essential. An authoritative product reference book should be kept available in the reception area, to help staff answer any queries a client may have. The book should contain information on what specific essential oils can be used for, how they should be diluted and contra-indications.

The general ambience of the salon is important in terms of making clients feel welcome and relaxed. Essential oils diffused in the reception area can greatly enhance the atmosphere of the salon and help towards sales potential. Other possible features, recommended by Feng Shui practitioners, and complementary to aromatherapy treatments, include relaxing music, a small water fountain and green foliage plants.

HEALTH AND SAFETY
If an essential oil or aromatherapy product accidentally splashes in a client's eye, steps must be taken to wash out the eye. Pre-prepared, sterile eye washes are available from good chemists, or first aid services such as the St John's Ambulance Brigade.

As a precautionary measure, all salons offering aromatherapy treatments should have an eye-wash in their first-aid kit. At the very least, an eye bath and distilled water should be readily available.

Aromatherapy Clients

Clients who have essential oil facial or body treatments may have asked their therapist's advice on what products they can use at home. This may be related to the treatment given, or it may be for more general use – such as to relax in the evenings. Whatever the purpose of the product, a note should be made on the client sheet, detailing what was bought. The purpose of this is so that, on the next visit, the therapist can enquire how effective the client found the product. If the therapist knows what products the client already has at home, she may be able to suggest another product to complement it.

Display of Essential Oils and Aromatherapy Products

Essential oils can degrade if left in sunlight, or near heat sources such as radiators, central heating ducts, warm pipes or light bulbs. Essential oils and aromatherapy products should therefore be displayed away from exposure to sunlight, towards the back of the reception area. (See *Health and Safety* box left, as essential oils are also flammable.)

Essential Oils for Sale

It is important to only sell essential oils that are suitable for home use, and tester bottles could be made available. The range should include those with no toxicological possibilities, which are safe for use in pregnancy, on children and for general home care. A basic range could include:

camomile roman	*mandarin*
eucalyptus	*palmarosa*
geranium	*rose*
jasmine	*rosemary*
lavender	*sandalwood*
lemon	*tea tree*

It is only necessary to offer for sale one base vegetable oil, in which the essential oils can be diluted by the client. *Sweet almond oil* is the best oil for this purpose, as it can be used on both face and body, and is suitable for all skin types.

There is no need to sell a variety of vegetable oils, as the blending of these base or carrier oils is a specialist subject, and the province of the aromatherapist.

Other Aromatherapy Products

The salon may wish to pre-prepare products for retail sale. Different products could be prepared for the different skin types, and could include:

bath lotions	*face oils*
body lotions	*moisturisers*
body oils	*sprays*
cleansers	*tonics*
face creams	

TIP

Although essential oils and aromatherapy products cannot be displayed in salon windows, empty bottles and containers can.

HEALTH AND SAFETY

Essential oils are flammable, which means they have a flash-point and can ignite if left near heat sources.

Care must be taken to ensure that essential oils are not stored near any form of heat, including sunlight.

These products should be well-displayed, making a feature of them. Leaflets describing the product, including instructions as to their use, can be given to the purchasing clients. These leaflets could also provide information on the other aromatherapy products on sale, as well as details about the treatments offered by the salon.

The laws pertaining to the retail sale of cosmetic or aromatherapy products are extensive, and discussed in *Essential Oils and Aromatherapy Products – The Law*.

Diffusing Essential Oils in the Reception Area

Gentle and relaxing blends of essential oils can be diffused in the reception area. These not only make the client feel more relaxed, but act as a subtle subconscious message that the client has entered a place of special pampering and luxury. The blends used can vary from time to time, or from season to season. Such blends should be prepared by an aromatherapist or staff-member with blending skills, or purchased from the many blends specialist companies have for retail sale.

The reception area diffuser blends of essential oils can also be offered for sale to clients. They may be a mix of two or more essential oils, and pre-prepared in small amber bottles. The bottles should be labelled, with details of their contents, and any details required by law.

> **TIP**
> Put a notice on the wall of the seating waiting area, advising clients that the diffuser blend being used that day is available for sale.

Smelling Strips to Maximise Sales

Paper smelling strips are a good way for a client to experience more closely the aroma of a certain essential oil or blend of oils. A supply of strips could be kept in the retail sales or reception area. A drop of essential oil is placed on the end of the strip, while the client holds the other end. The strip should be held about four inches under the nose, and turned in small circles, as the client inhales deeply.

Depending on the policy of the salon, clients can be invited to experience the aroma of individual essential oils or the various 'reception area diffuser blends'. If the client likes a particular fragrance, they can keep the smelling strip to place around the home or in a clothes drawer. If the aroma proves pleasing to the client, they may wish to purchase a bottle of that essential oil, or blend of oils, on their next visit.

Other Retail Possibilities

Essential oils are often used in diffusers. There are two main types: those powered by small, night-light candles, and those powered by electricity. Both require water to be placed in the bowl section, to which 6–8 drops of essential oil are added. Diffusers can be sold in the reception area, along with the essential oils.

When giving treatments using essential oils, any music played should be very relaxing. Many appropriate audio-tapes are available through specialist suppliers. These same tapes could also be sold at the reception area, to help clients re-create the special, relaxing atmosphere they find at the salon.

PURCHASING AND STORAGE OF ESSENTIAL OILS

Purchasing

When purchasing essential oils, several factors indicate that the supplier is responsible, and complying with the law as it affects them:

- Essential oils should be supplied in amber or dark-coloured glass, to prevent ultra-violet light penetrating the bottle. When sold in large quantities, essential oils are often packaged in bottles made of anodised aluminium, which have a thin coating of aluminium oxide – a good unreactive material.
- When essential oils come into contact with oxygen (or light), the double-bonds of the terpene components can break, leading to changes in the essential oil. For this reason, the containers in which the essential oils are supplied should be almost full, containing as little oxygen as possible.
- When purchasing large volume containers of essential oils, of 10 litres (2 gallons) or more, the following information should be available from the supplier if requested (EC Legislation 91/155/EEC):
  - the commercial name of the essential oil
  - the botanical nomenclature (Latin name)
  - main components (chemical composition)
  - any additives (carriers such as vegetable oil, alcohol or solvent; preservatives; or anti-oxidants)
  - potential health hazards (to skin or eyes; or when inhaled or ingested)
  - first-aid measures (relating to the above)
  - type of extinguishing media to use in case of fire (usually foam or carbon dioxide – do not use water)
  - spill and leak procedures (including environmental protection and cleaning methods)
  - handling and storage advice
  - protection methods for the individual handling essential oils
  - physio-chemical properties of the essential oil (including its colour; odour; pH value; boiling point; flash-point – the temperature at which it will automatically ignite; specific gravity; optical rotation; solubility in water; evaporation rate)
  - stability and reactivity (chemical stability; conditions to be avoided; hazardous decomposition products)
  - toxicological information (acute toxicity; dermal irritation; phototoxicity)

– eco-toxicological information (if toxic to bacteria and fish)
– recommended disposal method
– transport information (that may be required if being shipped elsewhere).

Suppliers who sell adulterated essential oils fall under the jurisdiction of the Trading Standards Department of your Local Authority.

Storage

The key points to remember when storing essential oils are that:

- their bottles or containers should always be kept tightly closed;

and they should be kept in a place that is:

- cool – away from heat sources;
- dark;
- dry – without humidity.

Light, like oxygen, can degrade essential oils, by breaking the double-bond terpene components. This can cause the essential oil to become sticky and resin-like, or a loss of quality due to the formation of peroxide radicals:

- When a large quantity of essential oil is taken into stock, a record should be kept of the date it was received. With larger bottles of essential oil, the delivery date can be written directly on the label.

In general, essential oils retain their therapeutic properties for up to one to two years. However, the citrus essential oils (lemon, lime, orange, grapefruit, mandarin, tangerine and yuzu) deteriorate more quickly than other essential oils, and have a therapeutic shelf-life of six months to one year. After this time their pleasant aromas continue, and can be used for fragrance-only purposes. To ensure that the essential oils you buy are effective, only purchase enough for 2–3 months' use, and re-order regularly.

ESSENTIAL OILS AND AROMATHERAPY PRODUCTS – THE LAW

If a salon intends to produce their own label cosmetic products, whether containing essential oils or not, they should refer to the *Cosmetic Products (Safety) Regulations 1996*, the European Directive 76/768/EEC, and other directives. A guide to these regulations should be available through your local library. Aromatherapy products fall within the scope of the *General Product Safety Regulations 1994 (Statutory Instrument 1994 No. 2328)*, available through your local library or The Stationery

Office (see Appendix at the end of this book), the Department of Trade and Industry's *A Guide to the Cosmetic Products (Safety) Regulations*, and other relevant literature.

Preparing Products for Individual Clients

A distinction is made in law between a product a therapist may prepare for the personal use of an individual client, and the marketing and sale to the public of cosmetic products. When a therapist prepares a product for an individual client, that does not come within the usual cosmetic regulations. However, a therapist should have product liability insurance if she intends to supply products to clients.

Selling Essential Oils

Although it is well known, and in many cases scientifically proven, that essential oils can have a direct beneficial effect upon health, it has become illegal to advertise or market an essential oil as a medicine unless a licence to do so has been granted by the European Commission. A customer might have been told, or read in a book, that a certain essential oil is helpful in treating a certain condition, and they are free to buy that essential oil. However, it is illegal for retail use labelling or packaging purposes to claim the essential oil can cure anything.

TIP

If manufacturing products for retail sale, whether containing essential oils or not, the salon management should designate a person to become thoroughly acquainted with the laws regarding cosmetic manufacture and marketing, to ensure the salon complies with them.

CHAPTER 7

Client Care

CLIENT ASSESSMENT

Assessment starts with the client being given a consultation form to fill in themselves. This is then used as a basis for discussion, within the verbal consultation, during which the therapist will make further notes on the form. A typical procedure follows this pattern:

- client completes initial consultation form;
- therapist consultation with the client;
- a detailed facial skin examination (if applicable);
- the first facial treatment (if applicable);
- the first body treatment (if applicable).

The purpose of these procedures is to ascertain:

- are there any contra-indications to treatment, or specific essential oils;
- treatment to be given.

The consultation should cover the six broad areas:

- basic personal information;
- medical history/medication;
- allergies;
- emotional state;
- lifestyle;
- diet.

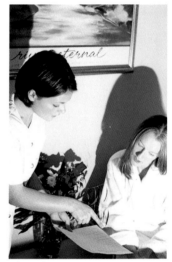

Client being given consultation form to complete

THE INITIAL CONSULTATION FORM

Salon Name, Address, Phone Number

PART 1:

Client's name: ....

Address: ....

....

Phone number(s): ....

Date of birth: ....

PART 2: Medical Details

General Practitioner's name: ....

Practice address: ....

Phone number: ....

Consultant's name: ....

Practice address: ....

Phone number: ....

Are you undergoing, or have you undergone, treatment for the following conditions?

Circulatory disorders: ....

High or low blood pressure: ....

Diagnosed heart condition: ....

Epilepsy: ....

Asthma: ....

Any serious illness or condition: ....

Frequent headaches or migraine: ....

Sinus problems: ....

Ear aches or infections: ....

Eczema or psoriasis; other skin conditions: ....

All current medications being taken: ....

Known allergens: ....

Diabetes: ....

Major surgical operations: ....

Accidents or fractures: ....

Any physical problems as yet undiagnosed: ....

Respiratory problems: ....

Rheumatism/Arthritis: ....

This section need only be completed if the client is having body treatment

---

Are you pregnant? .... Date due: ....

Menstrual problems: ....

Menopausal problems: ....

This section need only be completed if the client having body treatment is female

---

PART 3: Emotional Factors

Are you suffering from any of the following?

Stress: ....

Anxiety: ....

Depression: ....

PART 4:

Client's signature .... Date ....

Therapist's name: ....

This section must be completed by all clients

ADDITIONAL LIFESTYLE FORM

An additional lifestyle form is a helpful reference when the client is coming to the salon for a course of treatments. Suggested questions could include:

Do you smoke? (If yes, how many a day?)
Are you involved in any sports?
Do you take any other exercise?
Occupation:
  Do you work in a smoky atmosphere?
  Is there air conditioning/central heating?
  Do you work near electrical equipment?
  Are there chemicals in the atmosphere?
Do you have difficulty in sleeping?
How much fruit and vegetables do you eat per day?
How many caffeine drinks per day? (coffee, tea, coke)
How much alcohol do you drink a week?
How much water do you drink per day?

THERAPIST'S CONSULTATION WITH THE CLIENT

When the client has completed the consultation form and, in some cases, the additional lifestyle form, the therapist should read the responses while sitting with the client. This gives the therapist the opportunity to discuss with the client any issues she may want to investigate further. At this time, the therapist can ask the client why she has requested essential oil treatment(s) – for example, to relax, increase energy or just to feel pampered.

THE FACIAL SKIN EXAMINATION

As well as determining whether the client's skin is dry or dehydrated, for example, a thorough skin examination will determine many other factors. As you examine the face, you may consider whether particular areas require different treatments.

As well as the face itself, examine the neck and décolleté, and when answering these questions, make a note of which areas are affected:

- What is the general skin tone?
- Does the skin appear slack?
- Do the muscles lack tone?
- Is there tension being held in the muscles?
- Does the skin appear hydrated or dehydrated?
- Are there any nodules or swelling?
- Are there any broken capillaries?
- Are there areas of excessive oiliness?
- Are there dry or flaking patches?
- Are there open pores?
- If there are lines, are they light or deep?
- Is there excessive redness?
- Does the skin have a healthy appearance, or a greyish or sallow tone?

- Is there sun damage?
- Are there signs of cosmetic surgery?
- Are there any swollen lymph?
- Does the sinus area feel thick and congested?

MEDICATIONS AND THEIR EFFECTS ON THE SKIN

The reason this chart has been included is because often a client has a skin complaint that is not caused by internal physical or emotional factors, but by an adverse reaction to the use of a prescribed drug for a particular condition. The therapist confronted with such a condition will not be able to treat it, as the source of the problem is continuing with the use of the prescribed drug. The therapist could suggest to the client that they speak to their general practitioner or consultant to see if an alternative prescribed drug could be offered.

Many common drugs can have side-effects on the skin. The following chart shows the generic name of a drug, which may be included in several brand-named pharmaceutical products. For example, benzoyl peroxide, which is the most commonly prescribed drug for acne and fungal infections, is found in the pharmaceutical products which are marketed under the names *Acetoxyl, Acnecide, Acnegel, Benoxyl, Nericur* and *Panoxyl*. In addition, it is included in the combined preparations *Ancidazil, Benzamycin, Quinoderm* and *Quinoped*. All these products have the potential to cause the side-effects shown for benzoyl peroxide.

MEDICATIONS AND THEIR POTENTIAL SIDE-EFFECTS ON THE SKIN

★ = Common
■ = Rare

	Rash	Itching	Stinging	Burning Sensation	Redness	Flushing	Acne	Peeling	Dry Skin	Oily Skin	Blistering	Crusting	Swelling	Skin Changes	Skin Irritation	Soreness
Aciclovir	■	★	★	★												
Allopurinol	★	★														
Amoxycillin	★	■														
Atropine	★					★			★							
Beclomethasone ointment														★		
Bendrofluazide	★															
Benzoyl Peroxide			★		★			★	★		■	■	■		★	
Calcipotriol	■														★	
Captopril	★															
Clotrimazole	■		★	★											■	
Co-Trimoxazole	★	★														
Danazol							★			★						
Dithranol	■			★	★										★	
Dydrogesterone	★															
Erythromycin	★	★														
Fenbufen	★															
Fluticasone ointment														★		
Glyceryl Trinitrate						★										
Gliclazide	■	■				★										
Hydrocortisone						★										
Isosorbide Dinitrate/ Mononitrate						★										
Lamotrigine	★															
Lofepramine						★										
Methoxsalen					★											★
Nicorandil						★										
Nicotinic Acid	■	■				★										
Nifedipine						★										
Penicillamine	★	★														
Prednisolone							★									
Propylthiouracil	★	★														
Sodium Aurothiomalate	★	★														

The information in this chart is extracted from *The British Medical Association New Guide to Medicines and Drugs, 1997* (London: Dorling Kindersley).

CHAPTER 8

Aromatherapy for Facial Treatments

TIP

It is always preferable to use entirely natural ingredients as mediums in which to dilute essential oils.

TIP

A younger client will respond more quickly to treatment than an older person. Also, the speed of treatment will be affected by the amount of fluid congestion or fat in the facial tissue.

TIP

The production of the skin's natural moisturiser, sebum, is influenced by hormones. As certain essential oils may influence the hormonal level, a mixture of suitable essential oils and vegetable oil are one of the best ways to treat skin problems that are caused by hormonal imbalances. Refer to the individual essential oil and vegetable oil profiles.

Aromatherapy facials have become very popular because both client and therapist can see immediate results, with the skin looking refreshed and more dynamic, while the features are more relaxed because the client feels less stress and tension. The treatment also gives the client an overall sense of well-being. Essential oils or hydrolats are used in facial treatments in several forms including:

- **cleansers**
- **tonics**
- **massage oils**
- **face masks**
- **compresses**
- **poultices**
- **steaming**
- **eye pads**
- **moisturisers**

If the essential oils are pure and still therapeutically active, in addition to having an effect on the face, they will also have an effect on the body – through inhalation, and absorption through the dermis. Eventually, minute amounts of the aromatic components enter the bloodsteam. Experience shows that blood circulation and lymphatic flow seem to be made more efficient by the use of essential oils, and these are certainly means by which the skin can be improved.

Because essential oils have such excellent permeability (they penetrate the skin and tissues of the body very quickly), scientists around the world have been looking into the possibility of using them as a delivery system for medications. This is called 'the piggy-back effect'. Clearly, the permeability of essential oils is one reason why they are so effective as a beauty therapy treatment. However, it is important not to mix essential oils into products that contain any synthetic components, as these might inadvertently be carried into the body by 'piggy-backing' on to the essential oils which permeate the skin with such ease.

PRIOR TO TREATMENT: CONSULTATION AND SKIN EXAMINATION

Before commencing the first treatment, a full consultation and skin examination should be given. Refer to Chapter Seven, and follow the procedures outlined there. The first facial treatment must be thought of as part of the consultation process, and explained to the client as such. It will enable the therapist to ascertain factors that are not always apparent until the hands have been applied to the face during the course of treatment. After the first facial has been completed, successive treatments can be planned.

The initial consultation, and on-going consultations, give the beauty therapist the opportunity to find out exactly what improvements the client wishes to be achieved. Where do they wish to see changes first and foremost, and as time goes on?

DILUTING ESSENTIAL OILS FOR FACIAL TREATMENTS

Essential oils should always be diluted before application to the face, neck and décolleté area. In salon retail products, the percentage of essential oil included in the ingredients is likely to be between $1/8$ and 1 per cent of the whole. And with products intended for use on sensitive skin, the percentage is liable to be even lower.

The difference between the percentage of essential oil used in these day-to-day products, and the percentage of essential oil used in professional salon treatments, is often considerable. Professional aromatherapy facial treatments may have a higher percentage of essential oil for the following reasons:

- The application will be applied to the face for a maximum of 30 minutes at each session.
- Application is not daily. Depending on the condition being treated, the sessions will be spaced at 7–14-day intervals, for a series of 6–10 treatments.
- If a skin condition is being treated, it often responds well to higher volumes of essential oils, at the initial stage.

Using correct procedure within the salon environment, skin responds very well to the use of higher percentages of essential oils. The client and beauty therapist can see an immediate difference in the skin, which is evident for a week or more after treatment.

THE PERCENTAGE VOLUME OF ESSENTIAL OIL TO USE

Even if the treatment being given is the same, the percentage of essential oil used in a facial will vary from client to client, unless pre-packaged products are used. This variability is dependent upon the client's skin type, tone and sensitivity; their emotional state including stress and tension; any allergies or medical skin conditions; whether the client is taking medication or other

THE PSYCHOLOGICAL BENEFITS OF ESSENTIAL OILS

In general, the essential oils chosen for the face should have a relaxing and calming effect on the client. The psychological benefits of essential oils can be more fully realised during a facial in the salon environment because:

- the aroma molecules are inhaled constantly during a facial, because of the proximity of the nose;
- the aroma molecules are more concentrated in the atmosphere of an enclosed salon room or cubicle than when distributed throughout the air of a larger room in the home;
- the salon provides an atmosphere of relaxation, when the client can fully concentrate on themselves.

PARTIAL TREATMENTS

Depending on the policy of the salon, it may be possible to offer a client a partial treatment. Partial treatments are when treatments are applied to a specific area of the face or body that is causing concern – because it is blemished or scarred, for example.

If the client is coming to the salon for a facial, and yet there is a small problematic area on the body, it may be possible to apply aromatherapy beauty therapy techniques to that small area of the body, in addition to performing the facial.

drugs, undergoing radiation or chemotherapy treatment; and whether the client is pregnant. Each of these factors determines what volume of essential oil can be used. Such factors cannot be calculated for in a general retail sale product.

Skin Types

In the salon environment, skin which falls into the categories of normal, dry, oily, combination, problem, mature or dehydrated can be treated with a percentage of between 1–2½ per cent.

Skin Sensitivity

Until the skin's degree of sensitivity to the essential oils being used in the facial can be determined, use between ½–1 per cent.

Sensitive Skins

Carry out a patch test 24 hours before performing the treatment. Use between ½–1 per cent.

Acne

Skin with acne needs to be treated very gently, particularly if harsh commercial and prescription products have previously been used and have not been found helpful. The percentage of essential oil used will depend on the type and severity of the acne being treated, varying between 2 and 3 per cent.

Emotional State

On clients who are stressed and tense, and depending on the skin condition being treated, use between 2 and 3 per cent.

Depression

It is important to be aware of the possible side-effects of the medications for this condition. These can range from slight skin redness to a severe allergic reaction resulting in a burnt, scabbing appearance. If these are noticed, avoid using any essential oils on the client and refer them to their GP for advice. Otherwise follow the recommendations below in *Medications*.

Allergies

This refers to clients who suffer allergic reactions to foods or beauty products: until any allergic reaction to the treatment can be determined, use ¼–1 per cent.

- If the client is allergic to nuts, avoid using nut-derived oils in carrier or base oils.

Medications

It is possible the client's skin condition is a direct result of their medication. First refer to the medication skin side-effect list on page 98, and follow the procedures outlined there. In general, for people on medication use between $1/2$ and 1 per cent.

Undergoing Radiation or Chemotherapy Treatment

Often a person who is undergoing radiation or chemotherapy treatment, or has just finished such treatment, will visit a beauty therapist as a result of having developed skin conditions. Do not use essential oils or aromatherapy products at this time, unless it is a product especially designed for these clients.

Pregnancy

Refer to the list on page 11 for essential oils that cannot be used during pregnancy. The woman's hormonal and physiological changes must be taken into consideration. After careful choice of essential oils, use between $1/2$–1 per cent.

VEGETABLE OIL STARTER KIT

Choosing the correct vegetable oil(s) is as important as choosing the correct essential oils. Certain vegetable oils are often added in very small quantities, and even these small amounts can have a great therapeutic influence on the blends (for example: evening primrose, borage seed, red carrot root extract, jojoba, avocado and wheatgerm).

Vegetable oils such as camellia oil, jojoba and macadamia contain components that are very similar to those found naturally in the skin. Also vegetable oils rich in triple unsaturated fatty acids (such as wheatgerm, avocado, jojoba and hazelnut) not only help in maintaining the elasticity and tone of the skin, but strengthen the underlying connective tissue as well.

Which vegetable oils are chosen will depend on the client's skin type and condition and can be blended to suit the individual requirements of the client. The following would provide a good starter kit:

> **VEGETABLE OILS STARTER KIT**
>
> Sweet Almond Oil
> Hazelnut Oil
> Macadamia Oil
> Apricot Kernel Oil
> Avocado Oil
>
> The following should be used in small amounts, depending on the skin condition:
>
> Camellia oil, Rose-hip Seed oil, Jojoba oil, Red Carrot extract, Evening Primrose oil

SPECIALISED ESSENTIAL OIL FACIAL TREATMENTS
Tonics

Tonics are often applied after cleansing for their skin-enhancing effects. Their main role is to help remove any traces of the cleanser, and prepare the skin for other cosmetic preparations, although they can be applied for other purposes.

Tonics that are used after cleansing as part of an essential oil facial must be compatible with the essential oil massage oils. They would mainly consist of hydrolats or floral waters, or specialist toners for use before the application of essential oils.

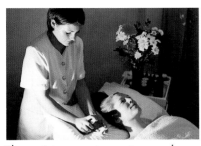
Therapist preparing cotton pad with tonic

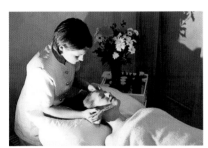
Applying face mask

Face Masks

All non-commercial face masks should be used as fresh as possible. The main ingredients can be made up and stored ready for when required, and then added to at the time of treatment. The main additions are hydrolats, herbal extracts and, of course, essential oils.

Steaming

If including steaming within a facial, only use the more gentle essential oils. Some steaming machines have been especially designed for use with essential oils, while essential oils are compatible with many machines that are not. Check with your steamer supplier if in any doubt. Although water and essential oils do not normally mix, the essential oils are made more volatile by the heat of steam, and the essential oil molecules rise with it. Use only small amounts of essential oil.

Poultices

Poultices are made by including a solid substance between layers of wet, hot or cold muslin. Ingredients used include herbs such as camomile, clays such as green clay, and crushed seeds such as linseed. Essential oils can be added to these.

Eye Pads

These are used for placing on the closed eyes, while the mask is taking effect. Eye pads can be soaked in an appropriate hydrolat. Good suggestions would be rose-water, eyebright, camomile and lavender.

Herbal or Floral Tea Compresses

A compress is a piece of natural material such as muslin that has been pre-cut into a round face-shape, with holes for the eyes, nose and mouth. For the neck and décolleté area, the shape of the compress would be square, and larger. The compress is soaked in a herbal preparation, and then squeezed out before application to the face.

Herbal or floral tea compresses are often used in aromatherapy facial treatments because they help prepare the skin for the essential oil massage. They may be warm or cold, depending on the desired result:

- Warm compresses allow blood to flow freely to the area, and for the pores to be gently opened. They can be very relaxing and calming, and are often used both before and after a treatment to help the absorption of the essential oils being used.

- Cold compresses are refreshing and somewhat restrict the flow of blood to the area. They are usually used after a treatment, especially if there is an inflammation or make-up is to be applied to the face.

Method

1. Make the liquid infusion by placing one teaspoon of the appropriate herb or flowers in a bowl or cup, and covering with hot water. Leave for some minutes, so the herb can 'brew' or steep, and cool down to the appropriate temperature.
2. Take the pre-cut piece of muslin and soak it in the herbal or floral infusion.
3. Let the muslin soak, then squeeze out the excess liquid.
4. While still wet, place the muslin over the face (or neck and décolleté).
5. Leave for one minute.
6. Remove the muslin, and pat the face dry with a clean paper tissue.
7. Wash or wipe hands to remove all traces of product before continuing with the treatment.

COMPRESS PLANT USES

★ Appropriate for skin type: COMPRESS PLANT	Sensitive	Dry	Normal	Oily	Acne	Rosacea	Mature	Revitalising
Arnica			★	★				
Bladderwrack	★			★				
Borage	★	★					★	★
Calendula/Marigold	★	★		★	★		★	
Camomile German	★				★	★		
Camomile Roman	★	★	★		★	★		
Caraway Seeds			★	★			★	★
Elderflower (flowers)	★	★						
Jasmine	★	★		★			★	★
Lavender	★		★	★	★	★		
Limeflowers	★	★					★	
Marshmallow	★	★					★	
Melissa			★	★	★			★
Oat	★	★		★				
Neroli			★				★	★
Peppermint				★	★			★
Rose Petals		★	★	★			★	★
Rosehip	★	★	★	★			★	★
Rosemary			★	★	★			
Sage		★	★	★	★		★	
St John's Wort	★	★			★	★		
Tea-Green, Camilla sinensis		★	★				★	★
Thyme				★	★			
Yarrow	★			★	★	★		

FACIAL REFLEX POINTS

Pressing reflex points as part of a facial increases energy flow, and leads to revitalisation.

The following movements are best carried out at the end of a facial:

- Press each of the points in sequence, for a few seconds each. Each point is approximately 1 centimetre ($\frac{1}{2}$ inch) apart. The movement is a gentle press and lift, then release.
- Do both sides of the face at the same time.
- The first movement involves pressing in a continuous line.

1. Start on the bridge of the nose, between the eyes, at the bottom of the forehead. Stroke in a continuous line straight up, to the centre of the hair-line. Use both thumbs, one following the other. Repeat several times.

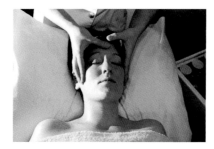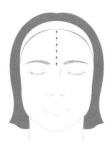

2. Start above the eyebrows, at the centre of the face. Press along the line of the eyebrows. Again, at the centre, move up about $^3/_4$ of a centimetre, and repeat the movement, working outwards. Carry on in this manner, until the whole forehead has been covered.

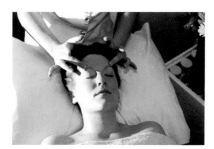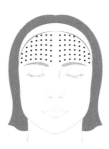

3. Smooth out both sides of the forehead, using all the fingers of both hands. Start at the centre, and smooth outwards towards the temples.

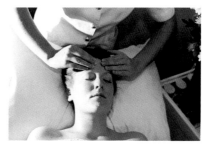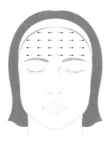

4. Place both hands on the forehead, and hold for a count of six.

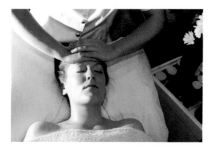

5. Starting under the inner eyebrows, press in a line working outwards.

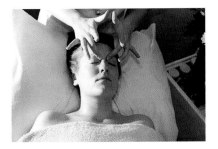 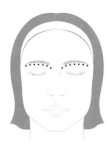

6. Press adjacent to the outer corner of the eyes.

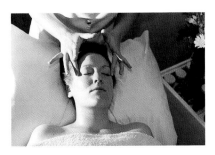 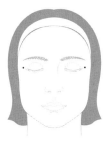

7. Starting either side of the bulbous part of the nose, work outwards towards the ear. This first line should be under the cheekbone. Repeat, moving upwards until the whole of the upper cheek is covered.

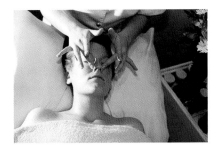 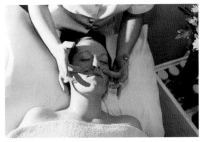 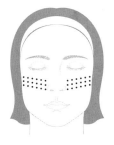

8. Smooth over the upper cheekbone, then the lower cheekbone. Work from the centre, outwards. Both movements should end at the temples.

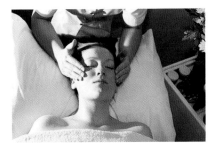

9. Starting above the side of the mouth, press in a line, outwards under the cheekbone. These points will involve lifting the flesh, and touching the cheekbone. Finish at the ear lobe.

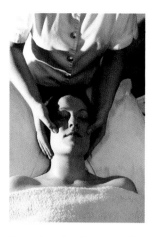 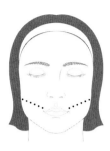

10. Starting in the area between the nose and upper lip, use two fingers to press outwards in a continuous line. Repeat several times.

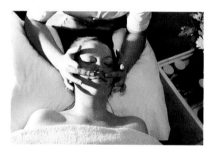 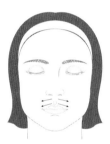

11. Starting under the lower lip, use two fingers to press outwards in a continuous line. Repeat several times.

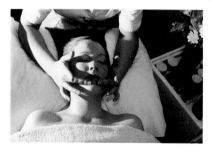 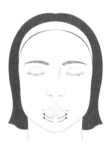

12. Pinch gently along the jaw-line, working outwards.

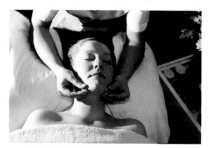 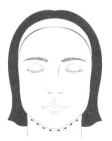

13. Press along the entire hair-line, starting at the middle and working towards the ear. Repeat several times.

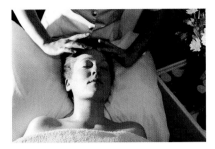
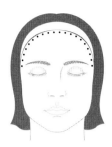

14. Using both hands, smooth upwards over both sides of the face, then over the forehead, up both sides of the neck and into a classic shoulder and neck finish.

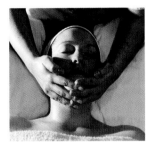
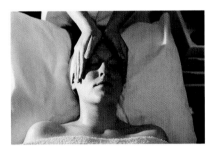
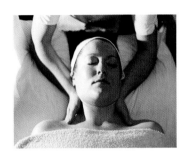

EXTRA REFLEX POINTS

These points can be inserted at any time while performing a facial massage. All help to improve the circulation and energy flow in the face, and also the tone of the skin. Hold each point for five seconds.

1. Both sides:
at centre of lower cheekbone
Use if the face looks tired or is sagging.

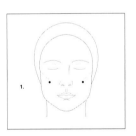

2. Both sides:
either side of the nose, in line with the inner corners of the eyes
Helps reduce sinus problems, and puffy eyes.

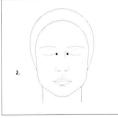

3. Both sides:
at the outer corners of the eyes
Use if the face looks tired or is sagging.

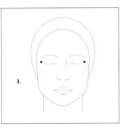

4. Third eye – in the middle of the eyebrows
Encourages bodily energy flow and calmness.

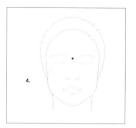

5. Both sides:
in the hollows just below the ears
Helps droopy cheeks and jowels.

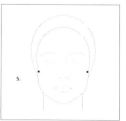

6. Both sides:
on the border between the eye sockets and cheek bones, in the middle
Helps to tone cheek muscles and lift the face. Reduces eye bags.

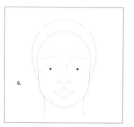

7. Both hands:
at the centre of the palms of the hands
Generally energises the whole body.

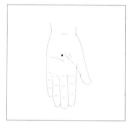

FACIAL MASSAGE WITH ESSENTIAL OILS

Massage is just one aspect of an essential oil facial treatment. It is carried out alongside the application of masks, poultices and compresses. Massage of the face, neck and décolleté area is beneficial for several reasons:

- it stimulates the blood supply in the area, which increases the oxygen level and improves the tone of the skin;
- the increased circulatory flow and the warmth created in the dermis by the massage movements allow for greater absorption of the essential oils;
- it relaxes facial muscle tension, softening the facial expression – is especially evident if the client is under stress, or with the more mature client;
- using drainage techniques stimulates the lymphatic flow in the area, which can help speed up the elimination of waste cellular matter, toxins and other impurities such as pollution;
- facial massage can help dispel tiredness, leaving the client feeling refreshed and relaxed.

Timing and Technique

- The facial massage itself should be no longer than a maximum of 20 minutes, and is more often between 10 and 15 minutes.

- The massage movement should be light but positive. The precise pressure used will very much depend on the skin type – such as sensitive or allergenic.
- In aesthetic aromatherapy, repetition of massage movements is known to have a very relaxing effect. For rhythm, and a memory connection to be made, each massage movement should be carried out between 4 and 6 times, depending on the skin type, age of the client and the treatment being performed.
- The beauty therapist must concentrate fully on the client, and the movements being performed during the massage. This assists the energetic flow from the hands, to the client. Hands should always be relaxed and the massage gentle, professionally flowing from one movement into another while melting away tense muscles.

BASIC ESSENTIAL OIL FACIAL MASSAGE

This facial massage includes reflex points, holding movements, light effleurage and deeper tissue work, and is carried out on the neck and shoulders, as well as the face. Work on both sides of the face at the same time.

1. First, warm your hands by rubbing them together using light friction, and imagining warm energy flowing into them. This will help warm the massage oil.
2. Pour a little of massage oil into the palm of one hand, and rub both hands together so the palms are covered with it.
3. Gently press the oil on to the face, starting at the chin and working up the face in sections towards the forehead.
4. Gently place your hands on the trapezius muscle and in a continuous, flowing movement using long strokes, move towards the occipital bone. Start with the right hand, followed by the left hand. Repeat six times. (The sweeping neck movements start the relaxation process, while some of the oil can penetrate the epidermis.)

    Wipe your hands.

5. Pour a little of the massage oil into your hands and use light effleurage movements, working upwards over the face.
6. Starting at the middle of the sternum, use effleurage in a smooth movement towards the armpits, gradually moving upwards and outwards in sections until the clavicle is reached. Use small circular travelling movements with the middle finger, following the bone outwards towards the armpits.
7. Repeat these movements on the upper side of the clavicle, following the bone. Finish this movement by placing your hands on both shoulders and remaining still for five seconds.
8. Return to the face, and use effleurage movements.
9. Starting at the centre of the chin, work upwards and outwards with your fingertips, following the mandible, until the ear is reached. Use firm but gentle, small-circular, stationary movements.

10. Move up approximately one centimetre (½ inch), and repeat the movements. Do this until the whole area under the lower lip is covered.
11. Starting at the centre of the upper lip, work outwards with your index fingertip, finishing at the ear. Use gentle pressure, small-circular, stationary movements, edging along one centimetre at a time. This is a repeating press-and-release movement. Moving upwards, repeat until underneath the cheekbone.
12. Take the cheek muscles between your thumbs and index fingers, and gently squeeze.
13. Rest for five seconds, resting both hands on the face. This movement aids energy-flow.
14. If incorporating reflex points into the massage, do so at this point. Refer to the instructions starting on page 105.
15. Smooth upwards along the sides of the face, starting at the chin and ending at the temples. Repeat three times. Then smooth the forehead, towards the ears.
16. Harmonise energy by holding the face in both hands for a few seconds.
17. Sweeping effleurage movements over the shoulders and neck. Repeat three times.
18. Extra product application:
    It is at this point that any essential oil concentrate can be used. If treating conditions such as acne or sensitive skin, a compress or poultice may be needed.
    Concentrate: apply gently and leave for the specified time.
    Compress: leave for between 1 and 3 minutes.
    Poultice: 5 minutes.
19. While your chosen extra product is left on the face, prepare a face mask.
20. Apply the mask. Leave it on the face for no longer than ten minutes.
21. Remove the mask and apply a compatible moisturiser.
22. Place both hands on the shoulders in the energy harmony position, to a count of six.
23. Leave the client to relax for a few minutes, then sit them up and give them a glass of water to drink.
24. To complete the treatment, rub your hand briskly but gently up the vertebrae.

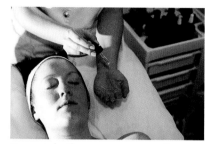

Essential oil concentrate application

This is a basic relaxing, yet facially energising essential oil treatment. There are many other techniques, which require hands-on training and cannot be adequately described in a book.

PERFORMING AN ESSENTIAL OIL FACIAL

- A facial using essential oils follows a pattern that is best suited to the absorption of those essential oils within the treatment time.
- The movements used are often very simple, with the emphasis on repetition, which has a very relaxing effect. Each movement is carried out between 4 and 6 times,

HEALTH AND SAFETY
If the client has been, or is currently on, a lot of medication, only use light, gentle movements during the first few facial treatments. This is because too much tissue stimulation and drainage at this stage may increase the movement of toxins in the bloodstream and produce headaches or nausea.

depending on the skin type, age of the client and the particular treatment being performed. The combination of essential oil products and repeated rhythmical movements creates a cellular memory effect.

- Essential oils also have a profound effect on the mind and emotional memory. Using movements which enhance the relaxing effect, in conjunction with essential oil products, allows for better absorption. The combination or synergy of mental/emotional and physical effects of essential oils creates an experience for the client unlike any other facial treatment.
- The results are visible, while the physical and emotional effects are felt immediately by the client, and the whole treatment will continue to work for up to 24 hours.

Time Required

First Appointment: 30 minutes verbal consultation; plus 1 hour observational treatment.
Subsequent Appointments: 1 hour.

The Treatment

An aromatherapy facial consists of the following steps:

1. cleansing;
2. natural refreshing tonic;
3. herbal compress;
4. essential oil massage;
5. application of compress or poultice;
6. facial mask;
7. application of moisturiser;
8. rest.

1. Cleansing

The main task of a cleanser is to thoroughly remove from the skin all traces of make-up and other facial products, and general dirt and grime.

When using essential oils in a facial treatment, cleansing is especially important because certain essential oil components have the capacity not only to penetrate the epidermis and dermis and enter the bloodstream, but also to act as a mode of transport for other substances.

The lipid attraction of the essential oil components is a unique feature, and makes it possible for essential oils to be diffused throughout the whole body. Not all substances can successfully attach to the essential oil molecules that enter the dermis in this way, but some can. If there is a substance on the surface of the skin that has the ability to attach itself to an essential oil molecule, that too may enter the epidermis and be transported into at least the upper layers of the dermis.

Using the correct cleanser and cleansing routine is thus of the utmost importance. Even the cleanest-looking skins need cleansing. Pollution is found on all skins. It comes from walking or driving along any road in any city. And in the countryside, where vehicle pollution is less, other hazards come in the form of air-borne pesticides, insecticides, fertilisers and growth enhancers – all of which can attach to the skin, and must be removed before treatment.

Cleansing Products

The cleansing product used must be one that has been specifically designed for use with, or be compatible with the use of, essential oils. It should be as natural as possible, and be free of synthetic chemical ingredients, additives and preservatives. It needs to have a gentle cleansing action and be easily removable. A cleanser that fulfils all these requirements would be equally appropriate for an oily or sensitive skin.

Vegetable Oils as Cleansers

Unrefined, organic vegetable oils can be used as cleansers. All are gentle on the skin, and some are particularly cleansing. Jojoba oil, for example, is not only a good facial cleanser, but can even be used to remove eye make-up.

As with all cleansers, vegetable oils will need to be removed by wiping the skin with a tonic or hydrolat, or by using a cloth dampened with water. Acned and problem skins often benefit from vegetable oil cleansers, which are also particularly effective for drying or ageing skins.

The Cleansing Routine

Most of the usual cleansing routines can be used:

1. First gently apply the cleanser over the face and throat area, gently loosening any make-up or grime.
2. Remove the cleanser, then wipe over the face with water, using a soft cloth, and repeat as needed.
3. Apply the cleanser over the décolleté, and the back of the neck area. Remove the cleanser with the toner.
4. Once the grime on the skin has been cleaned, a massage cleansing routine can be applied if necessary

2. Tonics

Remove all traces of the cleansing product using a natural tonic, hydrolat or floral water.

3. Herbal Tea Compresses

If using a herbal tea compress, this is the stage at which is will be applied.

4. Essential Oil Facial Massage

Choosing the Essential Oils and Base Oils

1. Prepare your base oil, having first consulted the base oil profiles for an appropriate choice, based on your client's skin type and the condition of their skin.
2. Choose your essential oil(s), considering the client's skin type and condition, and the objective of the facial. This may be to treat a particular condition, to revitalise the face, to make the client feel refreshed and energised or, if the client suffers from stress, to use appropriate oils with relaxing properties.

5. Poultice or Compress

If using a poultice or compress, this is the stage at which it will be applied.

6. Facial Mask

If using a facial mask, this is the stage at which it will be applied.

7. Moisturiser

Use a pure natural moisturiser if available. There is no need to add essential oils to this, as sufficient will have been used during the treatment.

ALLERGIES

It is important that before giving any facial treatment with essential oils, all allergies have been discussed with the client. As this is part of the usual initial consultation procedure, any relevant notes should be easily available to see on the client record card.

Clients who are allergic to wheat should not be given facials that include wheatgerm oil as part of the base oil. Nut-based vegetable oils should not be used on clients who are allergic to nuts. As well as foods, a client may be allergic to perfumes, soaps, detergents, cosmetics and many other substances. Generally, these clients are allergic to the synthetic chemicals within these products.

Although clients who suffer from allergies can be treated with essential oils, a patch test should be carried out 24 hours beforehand, using the same essential oil blend as you plan to used in the treatment itself. Treating skin allergies is a specialised area and such clients would be better suited to being treated by clinical/medical aromatherapists.

MEDICAL SKIN CONDITIONS

It is not the place of the beauty therapist to treat medical skin conditions. Clients with such conditions should be seen by a qualified clinical aromatherapist. There are two exceptions to this rule – acne and rosacea – and these are discussed below.

TREATING SPOTS DURING A TREATMENT

1. If intending to use essential oils on spots or blemishes, apply before the last compress in the facial treatment.

2. Prepare a mix of 2 drops of carrot root oil, plus 1 drop of an appropriate essential oil. **Lavender** or **tea tree** would be appropriate options.

3. With a cotton bud, apply the essential oil mix directly on to the affected pore.

ACNE FACIAL TREATMENT

Acne is caused by an increase in androgen hormone activity, which stimulates the functioning of the sebaceous glands. Within the hair follicle, the shedding of dead skin cells causes blockages within the follicle, which becomes infected. An overgrowth of skin over the pores is another factor. The skin's normal covering of bacterium becomes more active, and multiply rapidly. Anti-bacterial products cause inflammation not only in the hair follicle but within the surrounding area also, causing the characteristic redness of acne.

Acne usually starts to develop around adolescence, in both males and females, and clears up after 5–10 years. In some older people, acne can sometimes develop spontaneously. The face is the usual site of acne, although it can also appear on the chest, neck, shoulders, back, scalp, legs and upper arms. Acne can consist of all or some of the following:

black-heads:	result when blocked matter in the pores has oxygenated, and turned black.
comedones:	caused by the pores becoming blocked with a mixture of sebum and dead skin cells.
nodules:	large, inflamed areas with a large amount of pus – which can lead to scar tissue being formed, and scarring.
papules:	inflamed areas usually with no degree of infected matter – appearing under the skin.
pustules:	contain pus and inflammation.
scarring/macules:	a result of the immune system response to the infected areas, caused by the skin attempting to repair itself as best it can; if skin is treated correctly at the outset of acne, scarring and pitting can often be avoided.
white-heads:	result when the pore has closed, trapping matter inside – when the sebaceous matter becomes infected, it causes inflammation within the surrounding tissues.

There is evidence that hormonal factors play a role in the development of acne. Stress too is a factor, as stress can cause the adrenal glands to be stimulated, leading to hormonal imbalances.

Medications

The usual treatments for acne are often the excessive use of antibiotics and harsh anti-bacterial products which are applied topically. Products containing up to 10 per cent Benzoyl peroxide can strip the skin of its naturally oily mantle, causing dry skin, and have side-effects including in some cases the development of contact dermatitis. Retin A can lead to redness and scaling of the skin, which can also become very sensitive to sunlight and commercial products. Steroid treatments, particularly if applied topically, can cause facial erythema.

Many pharmaceutical drugs can cause a response in the skin which has an appearance very similar to that of acne. Antibiotics, sulphonamoides, barbiturates and anti-rheumatic agents are amongst these. Some people who use drugs for recreational purposes are often prone to skin conditions such as acne.

Acne Treatment

1. Cleansing should consist of the product being smoothed over the face with a disposable fabric or a piece of cotton wool. The cleanser should contain an anti-inflammatory substance such as azulene – a natural derivative of camomile german.
2. Carefully wipe the cleanser off with an appropriate hydrolat – such as thyme, myrtle, lemongrass, lavender or camomile german. Use disposable fabric or a piece of cotton wool.
3. Repeat the whole cleansing process at least twice.
4. Apply a compress of green tea (*Camilla sinensis*), and leave on the face for five minutes.
5. Dry the face, then apply your blend of essential oil in the appropriate base oil. Gently press the oil on to the face, starting at the chin and working up the face in sections towards the forehead.
6. Over the top of the oil, apply a warm, damp, green tea muslin compress.
7. If there is no acne on the neck, gently place your hands on the trapezius muscle and in a continuous, flowing movement using long strokes, move towards the occipital. Start with the right hand, followed by the left hand. Repeat six times. (This sweeping neck movement starts the relaxation process, while some of the oil can penetrate the epidermis.) *Do not massage the face itself, as this may cause further inflammation.*
8. Carry out this movement if the acne is confined only to the face. Starting at the middle of the sternum, use effleurage in a smooth movement towards the armpits. Gradually work outwards in sections until the clavicle is reached. Use small circular travelling movements with the middle finger, following the bone outwards towards the armpits.
9. Continue with this movement if the acne is confined only to the face. Repeat the above movements on the upper side of the clavicle, following the bone. Finish by placing your hands on both shoulders and remaining still for five seconds.

    Wipe your hands thoroughly.

10. Use the reflex points, as shown in the diagrams starting on page 106. Start at the forehead.
11. Harmonise energy by holding the face in both hand for a few seconds.
12. Extra product application:
    If using a compress, leave for between 1 and 3 minutes.
    If using a poultice, leave for 5 minutes.
13. Apply the mask. Leave it on the face for no longer than 10 minutes.

14. Finish by wiping with a hydrolat. No substitute may be used.
15. Place both hands on the shoulders in the energy harmony position.
16. Leave the client to relax for a few minutes, then sit them up and give them a glass of water to drink.
17. To complete the treatment, rub your hand briskly but gently up the vertebrae.
18. Ask the client to leave their skin free of all products for at least 24 hours.

Treatment Plan

Further salon visits will be required. Female clients should try to plan their visits mid-way through their menstrual cycle.

Weeks 1 and 2 – two sessions
Weeks 3 and 4 – one session
Weeks 6, 9 and 13 – one session
Monthly thereafter until the condition has improved.

Home Care

The client should use a gentle cleanser, a hydrolat as a tonic, and a facial oil and moisturising cream at home. They should be asked to use no other products – including make-up foundation – for at least one month. This will be difficult for some clients, but it may shorten the time required to improve the condition.

Although foods such as chocolate are now not thought to be a trigger of acne, there can be no doubt that a lack of the essential vitamins and minerals found in correct nutrition will lead to the body being unable to cope and repair itself adequately. It is therefore advisable that clients with acne are directed towards eating a nutrient-packed, organic diet until the condition has been righted. They are advised to cut out red meat, alcohol and packaged foods, and to eat fish, chicken, fruit, vegetables and raw food such as salads. In addition, they could take vitamin C, multi-vitamin and zinc supplements.

ROSACEA FACIAL TREATMENT

Rosacea is a skin condition that is recognisable by pronounced redness or flushing of the skin, particularly on the forehead, the bridge of the nose and the cheeks. In severe cases it can extend over the whole face, neck and décolleté area. Papules and pustules may be present, but seborrhoea and comedones are not.

The homeostatic control of blood vessels supplying the pilosebacous follicles appears to be disturbed, leading to dilation of the vessels. Why this occurs is unknown. The mite *Demodex folliculorum* is found on the skin of rosacea sufferers, but whether this is a cause or an effect of the condition is under debate. In some cases, the rosacea has been triggered by overuse of corticosteroid creams prescribed for other skin conditions.

Rosacea often develops slowly, over months or even years, changing from an occasional passing flush to a more permanent condition. Middle-aged women are the most likely group to be affected. Clients with this conditions may find their skin has become very sensitive to light, and to most skin products.

Rosacea Treatment

When performing a facial on clients with rosacea, follow the steps for the facial treatment on page 111, but make the following changes to the routine:

- omit step 8;
- omit step 12;
- step 20: use no masks other than pure aloe vera water;
- step 21: apply azulene-containing essential oils in a suitable base.

Treatment Plan

Further salon visits will be required:

Weeks 1 and 2 – two sessions
Weeks 3 and 4 – one session
Weeks 6, 9 and 13 – one session
Monthly thereafter until the condition has improved.

Home Care

The client should use a gentle cleanser, a hydrolat as a tonic, and a facial oil and moisturising cream at home. They should be asked to use no other products – including make-up foundation – for at least one month. This will be difficult for some clients, but it may shorten the time required to improve the condition.

Facial Treatments	Normal skin	Dry skin	Oily skin	Combination skin	Sensitive skin	Flaking skin	Revitalisation	Ageing skin	Mature skin	Regenerative	Toning	Scarring	Capillaries	Congestion	Puffiness	Itchiness	Eczema	Psoriasis	Rash	Inflammation	Infection	Blemishes	Acne	Seborrhoea	Sluggish	Purifying	Sinus congestion
Bergamot			●																		●	●	●	●			
Bois de Rose	●	●		●	●	●	●	●	●	●		●		●						●							
Camomile German	●	●		●	●							●		●	●	●	●	●	●	●			●	●			
Camomile Roman	●	●	●	●	●								●	●		●	●	●	●	●							
Cedarwood	●		●	●								●				●	●		●				●	●	●		
Clary Sage	●	●						●	●			●											●				
Cypress			●	●							●		●	●									●	●			
Eucalyptus Radiata			●									●									●		●		●		●
Fennel	●		●	●			●		●		●																
Frankincense			●	●		●	●	●	●			●		●							●	●		●			●
Geranium	●	●		●	●	●	●	●	●		●	●	●	●		●				●			●		●		●
Jasmine	●					●	●					●															
Juniper														●	●	●	●	●	●	●			●		●		
Lavender	●	●		●	●							●				●	●	●	●	●		●	●	●			
Lemon	●		●								●		●	●							●	●	●		●	●	
Lemongrass			●																		●	●	●	●			
Mandarin	●		●	●							●																
Melissa			●				●														●		●			●	
Neroli		●		●		●	●	●	●	●		●				●							●				
Orange			●	●									●	●								●			●		
Palmarosa			●					●	●	●		●				●					●		●	●		●	
Patchouli	●		●	●						●	●			●							●	●	●				
Petitgrain			●					●	●		●										●	●			●		
Rose Maroc	●						●	●	●																		
Rose Otto	●	●	●		●	●	●	●		●		●	●														
Rosemary			●											●									●	●	●		●
Sandalwood	●	●		●	●			●	●		●				●				●	●			●				
Tea Tree																●		●	●		●		●	●			●
Thyme Linalol															●						●	●	●			●	
Vetiver			●					●	●		●											●	●				
Violet Leaf								●	●		●				●								●				
Ylang-ylang			●	●			●				●	●															

CHAPTER 9

Essential Oil Body Treatments

It is not the aim of this book to replace training in aromatherapy massage, but to explain more fully the use of essential oils during body treatments, along with movements and reflex points that can be incorporated into massage for the benefit and well-being of the client. There are many aromatherapy techniques that cannot be explained in a book, and a therapist must have hands-on experience to learn them.

Massage helps to increase circulation and oxygenation, stimulates the tissues, relaxes and tones the muscles, releases tension and increases lymphatic flow. It can help with the process of digestion, while stimulating the body to release and remove waste matter and toxins from the body.

There are many forms of massage and the type of movement used will depend on the result aimed for. A person may visit a beauty salon to have a full body massage, to relax, to ease aching muscles, or to carve a small amount of time out of their busy lives for themselves. Body massage treatments using essential oils can be for:

- slimming
- toning
- energising
- relaxing
- healing

The role of massage can be seen in several distinct ways:

- To reduce tension: a full body or back massage; neck and shoulder massage, or foot massage.
- As part of an inch-reduction treatment, with emphasis on a specific area.
- Lymphatic drainage massage aims to reduce oedema conditions and build-up of fluids.
- Massage incorporating acupressure/shiatzu/reflex points can treat specific conditions or help maintain good health and well-being.
- Sports massage techniques are used to tone, or release tension, from muscles; and in many cases to treat, or prevent, injuries.
- To give comfort in emotional crisis.

PRODUCTS

Therapists use a wide range of oil-based products which enable the hands to glide over the body effortlessly, including oils, lotions, creams and powders. Many commercially produced products state that they contain essential oils, when in reality they do not contain pure essential oils in sufficient quantity to deserve that description. However, using a therapeutic essential oil product intended for professional massage is a very different experience, and many beauty therapists are surprised at the pleasure they personally derive from using such products.

DILUTION OF ESSENTIAL OILS

The percentage of essential oils within a massage oil has been a controversial area of discussion within aromatherapy for many years. Aromatherapy books often suggest different dilution rates, which can be very confusing. The fact is that, scientifically, nobody can give a definite answer as to what an appropriate dosage should be, and there are no rules, only guidelines. The majority of scientific toxicology tests are carried out using undiluted essential oils. Dermatological sensitivity tests are carried out using various percentages of essential oil diluted in various mediums. The volumes of essential oil used in these tests are often extremely high in relation to body weight.

The scientific testing of essential oils is most often carried out for the cosmetic and perfume industry, who have to consider that their product is likely to be applied on a customer's skin every day, over a period of perhaps many years, in different climates and on different skins – including the most sensitive. The use of essential oils in aromatherapy or beauty therapy is very different. The client may be seen for an hour, once a week or once a month.

If essential oils adversely affected the health, full-time aromatherapists would be the first to suffer. However, this does not seem to be the case. Indeed, the early pioneers in this field are still extremely dynamic men and women, travelling all over the world to teach and lecture, long after many others of their generation have retired to their arm-chairs!

In beauty therapy treatments, it is always best to use less essential oil rather than more. Dosages should be appropriate for the treatment, and provide the service and result the client expects. Real essential oils, used in correct dosages, provide therapeutic activity and have a very real effect on the client's well-being.

BASIC RELAXING BODY MASSAGE USING ESSENTIAL OILS

Reflex Points for relaxation and toning

The following reflex points can be included during the massage treatment. As well as using finger-pressure, these points can be stimulated by the use of healing compresses and poultices, or by massage over the area.

TIP

All essential oils that are used on the face can be used on the body. But not all essential oils used on the body can be used on the face.

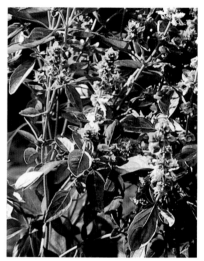

Sweet basil

PERCENTAGES OF ESSENTIAL OIL TO USE FOR BODY TREATMENT PURPOSES

Use the lower amount if the client has a sensitive skin, or is on medication, or is considerably biologically aged.

$1\frac{1}{2}$–2 per cent for general relaxation

2–$2\frac{1}{2}$ per cent body massage

3 per cent when treating a specific condition; or aches and pains; or during slimming, cellulite or toning treatments

Finger-pressure is applied by placing the middle finger over the index finger. Use the lower finger to massage the points, with small, stationary, circular movements. The word 'stationary' indicates that the fingertip doesn't move over the skin, but stays on one reflex point, moving in imperceptibly small circles. Pressure is applied for no more than three seconds each time. A natural rhythm will emerge, and it is possible to incorporate pressure of the reflex points within the flow of the massage. Effleurage can be applied between each pressure point.

1. On the sole of the foot: ³/₄ way down the foot, in line with the big toe joint Energises and stimulates the body.

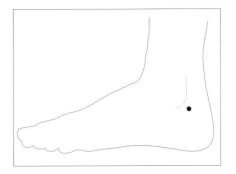

2. Just behind the ankle bone – on the outside of the foot

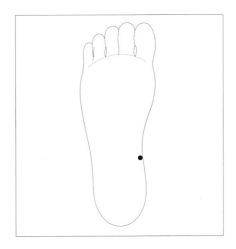

3. Under the ball of the foot

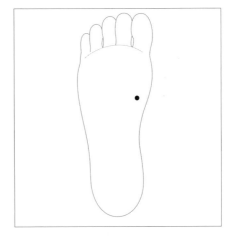

4. On the back: at the level of the waist line – 2 points, either side of the vertebrae

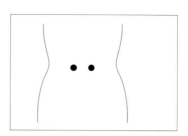

5. On the back: about 1 inch above the level of the waist line – 2 points, 2 inches away from the vertebrae

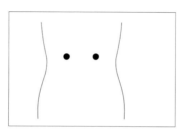

6. On the back: working up on either side of the vertebrae, to the shoulder blades

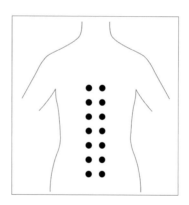

7. On the front: approximately 3 inches below the navel
Helps with weight reduction, cellulite, helping rid the system of impurities, improves circulation and reproductive system.

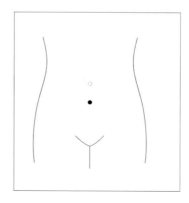

8. On the front: 1 inch either side of the navel (depending on the amount of fat accumulated in the belly area, for the therapist it is better to use two points $^{1}/_{2}$ an inch apart)
Overall energising; removing static in the abdominal area.

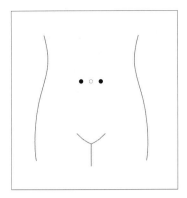

9. On the front: approximately 4 inches directly above the navel

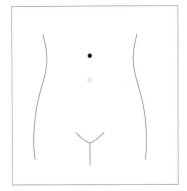

Preparing the Room

Before the client enters the treatment room, all basic preparations should have been carried out:

- The lighting should be dimmed.
- Not all clients like to hear music while having massage, and some appreciate total peace and quiet. Other clients may like to talk. Music is a very subjective experience, with personal taste being very varied. If using music in the treatment area, choose gentle, unobtrusive music that can suit most tastes. In general, instrumental music is more relaxing.

Equipment

- Two large towels, large enough to cover the whole body. Bath-size towels, or sheets, may be used. These are required to prevent the essential oil evaporating once massage in each area has been completed.
- Two body rolls, baby pillows or small towels that can be rolled up. These are for placing under the client's neck, shoulders, knees or ankles – wherever they are required to relieve pressure on certain areas of the body.

  To help support the breast, a small rolled towel or other support can be placed under the sternum. A soft pillow can be used for women with larger breasts, and those with upper back and shoulder pain.

Client Modesty

It is easier for the therapist if the client removes all clothing, but many clients find this embarrassing, and the removal of clothes must be the client's choice. Make this clear to the client at the outset.

Client Examination

Carry out the following examination:
Have the client sit on the couch with their back towards you.

1. Examine the vertebrae for any misalignments, redness or lumpiness.
2. Note the posture. Are they leaning forward with the head hung down? Are the shoulders rounded?
3. Smooth one hand over the whole of the back to feel how tense or stressed the muscles are. This will help in your choice of essential oils, and helps determine the bodywork technique that is required.

To further help you with your choice of essential oils and bodywork techniques, ask the client to lie on their front, and carry out a brief skin analysis.

4. *Pale skin* may indicate poor blood circulation or a medical condition such as anaemia or low blood pressure.
5. *Discoloured areas* may indicate toxicity or previous bruising.
6. *Yellowish skin or skin with poor pallor* may indicate kidney problems or liver conditions.
7. *Bluish tinge* may indicate poor blood circulation.
8. *Cold hands and feet* may indicate poor blood circulation.
9. *Varicose veins* may indicate colon problems, back problems, lack of exercise, stagnant energy and fluid flow.
10. *Spongy tissue* may indicate water retention or poor nutrition.
11. *Tension in the muscles* may be caused by injury, stress or holding the body in a fixed position.
12. *Knotted fibrous tissue* may indicate scar tissue or congestion.
13. *Hard and congested areas* may indicate crystallisation.
14. *Thickened toe nails* may indicate a fungal, rheumatic or arthritic condition.

Commencing Treatment

Back of the Body

Back: Before removing the towel, place one hand flat over T1, and the other over the sacrum area. Then remove the towel, apply the oil and commence the massage. Incorporate any of the reflex points outlined above if you feel they are appropriate. Finish by holding once again over T1 and the sacral area.

Legs and Feet: Remove the towel covering the legs, and use the hand holding positions – first on the soles of the feet, then behind the knees, then on the thighs. Pour a little oil into your hand and rub both hands together in a friction movement. Smooth over enough oil, and commence your leg massage. When you have finished, use the 1, 2 and 3 reflex points on both feet, before covering the legs with the towel.

Front of the Body

Legs and Feet: Repeat the leg holding and energising reflex point, as on the back of the body. Cover the legs.

Abdomen: Hold one hand over the lower abdomen, and the other hand over the chest area – covering the thymus gland. Start your massage by working on the abdominal area first, incorporating any front of the body reflex points that you feel to be appropriate. Cover the client's abdomen and breasts with a towel. Starting on the left side of the chest, and using a light effleurage movement – with one hand following on from the other in a continuous flowing movement, drain along the clavicle, into the armpit. Repeat the movement on the right side, and finish with general decollete effleurage movements used in Swedish massage, not forgetting to incorporate the shoulder area.

Arms: Press the reflex point at the centre of the hand (see page 110) for a count of three. To finish, use holding pressure on the inner arms – in three sections: lower arm, inner upper arm (just above the elbow), and inner arm just before the armpit. Repeat the draining movement before moving to the other arm.

Neck: Use gentle sweeping movements up the neck, to the base of the occipital. Then use small, circular travelling movements with three fingers, travelling in an upwards direction, either side of the cervical vertebrae. Starting once again on the left side of the chest, repeat the light continuous effleurage movement – one hand following on from the other, draining along the clavicle and into the armpit. Repeat on the right side. Effleurage around the shoulders and up the neck. Place the hands on the shoulders and hold for five seconds to finish.

VERTEBRAE AND NERVE CONNECTIONS

The back divides into five sections, with the nerves from all the organs and body areas connecting to a particular vertebra. Each vertebral section is also associated with a particular skeletal system.

During massage, use light, full-hand holding pressure over the indicated area, either side of the vertebrae, to help balance the flow of energy to that specified related area.

- *neck area* – cervical region: 7 vertebrae; 8 nerves
- *upper to mid-back area* – thoracic/dorsal region: 12 vertebrae; 12 nerves
- *mid to lower area* – lumber region: 5 vertebrae; 5 nerves
- *lower back, before buttock crease* – sacral region: sacrum vertebrae; 5 nerves
- *tail bone, coccyx* – coccygeal vertebra; 1 nerve

There are 12 pairs of cranial nerves and 31 pairs of other nerves, which extend from either side of the vertebrae:

Cervical Region

8 pairs of nerves.

C1	brain, pituitary gland, inner ear, head, scalp, bones of the face

Cervical spine
Seven vertebrae, the topmost of which supports the skull.

Thoracic spine
Twelve vertebrae that run down the rear wall of the chest. A pair of ribs is attached to each vertebrae.

Lumbar spine
Five vertebrae. This section is the one under the most pressure during lifting.

Sacrum
Five fused vertebrae.

Coccyx
Four fused vertebrae.

Vertebrae

	nerves to vertebral artery, eyes, throat, submandibular gland
C2	auditory, optic nerves, eyes, forehead, tongue, mastoid bone
	nerves to vertebral artery, larynx, eyes, sublingual gland
C3	trigeminal nerve (smell), cheeks, ears
	nerves to heart, lungs, diaphragm, vertebral artery
C4	eustachian tubes, lips, mouth, nose
	nerves to thyroid, diaphragm, vasomotor nerves, vertebral artery, trachea
C5	larynx, pharynx, vocal cords, neck glands
	nerves to thyroid gland, diaphragm, vertebral artery, trachea, oesophagus
C6	tonsils, neck and shoulder muscles
	nerves to vertebral artery, trachea, oesophagus, eyes, lungs, heart
C7	thyroid gland, arms
	nerves to vertebral artery, trachea, oesophagus, eyes, lungs
C8	eyes, lungs, trachea, bronchi, heart

Thoracic/Dorsal Region

12 pairs of nerves.

T/D1	oesophagus, trachea, lower arm
	nerves to eyes, ears, heart, lungs, pleura, vasomotor nerves, bronchi
T/D2	heart
	nerves to vasomotor nerves, intercostal nerves, pleura, heart, bronchi
T/D3	lungs, bronchial tract, breasts, chest
	nerves to intercostal nerves, pleura, heart, liver, diaphragm, bronchi
T/D4	gall bladder
	nerves to intercostal nerves, pleura, heart, lungs, diaphragm, trachea, mammary glands
T/D5	solar plexus, liver
	nerves to intercostal nerves, pleura, diaphragm, mammary glands, stomach, spleen, liver
T/D6	stomach
	nerves to intercostal nerves, pleura, diaphragm, stomach, spleen, liver
T/D7	pancreas, duodenum
	nerves to intercostal nerves, peritoneum, stomach, spleen, gall bladder, liver, pancreas
T/D8	spleen, diaphragm
	nerves to intercostal nerves, peritoneum, stomach, spleen, bile duct, gall bladder, pancreas, suprarenal glands
T/D9	adrenal glands
	nerves to intercostal nerves, vasomotor nerves, suprarenal glands, pancreas, small intestine

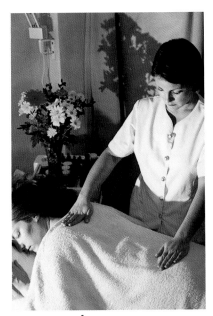
Energy transference

T/D10 kidneys
nerves to intercostal nerves, peritoneum, spleen, bile duct, diaphragm, urinary tract, kidneys, pancreas

T/D11 kidneys, ureter
nerves to peritoneum, diaphragm, urinary tract, small intestine, large intestine, pancreas

T/D12 small intestine, fallopian tubes
nerves to peritoneum, diaphragm, kidneys, urinary tract, small intestine, large intestine, appendix

Lumber Region

5 pairs of nerves.

L1 large intestine
nerves to small intestine, appendix, uterus, ovaries, fallopian tubes, testes, penis, bladder

L2 appendix, abdomen
nerves to large intestine, small intestine, appendix, uterus, testes, penis, ejaculatory duct

L3 ovaries, uterus, testes, bladder, knee
nerves to uterus, ovaries, fallopian tubes, prostate gland, ejaculatory duct, testes, penis, bladder

L4 prostate gland, sciatic nerve, lower back muscles
nerves to rectum, anus, prostate gland, bladder, uterus, sigmoid colon

L5 lower leg, ankle, feet, toes, arches
nerves to rectum, anus, prostate gland, bladder, uterus, sigmoid colon

Sacral Area

5 pairs of nerves.

genitalia, rectum, coccygeal gland, bladder, anus, erection, emission, vagina, cervix of the uterus

Coccyx

1 pair of nerves

coccyx coccygeal vertebra; 1 nerve

ENERGY TRANSFERENCE DURING MASSAGE

The human body functions on electromagnetic energy. Whenever a hands-on therapy such as body massage and facial massage are performed, an electrical exchange between therapist and client occurs naturally. Using essential oils heightens or amplifies this healing exchange.

It is wise to remember that electromagnetic exchanges work both ways and can affect the therapist, particularly if treating a person who is very tired. The therapist may find themselves feeling tired after performing a massage, while the client feels much refreshed. Learning not to allow a client to drain energy is very important if burn-out is to be prevented.

One of the techniques used to prevent energy drainage is visualisation. Visualise (or visually imagine) your own energy-flow circulating around your body without coming into contact with the client.

Healers, massage therapists and other body workers are trained in various techniques to prevent the loss of their own energy. Indeed, learning to conserve their own energy is the first step in training in those fields, because without it those practitioners would very soon burn out.

BLENDING FOR BODYWORK

Certain essential oils are automatically compatible with other essential oils. For example, one could use all stimulating essential oils in a blend, or essential oils that have calming or soothing properties in a relaxing blend.

Exceptions occur in medical aromatherapy or when treating a particular condition. For example, if you require a blend that it is both anti-inflammatory and energising, first identify in the essential oil profiles those that are anti-inflammatory, then look among those oils for ones which are also energising or stimulating. Also refer to the chart at the end of this chapter. If you find an essential oil or oils that fit both your requirements, use them. If not, use the least chemically stimulating essential oil from the stimulating oil list, to combine with the anti-inflammatory essential oils (refer to *The Chemistry of Essential Oils* in Chapter 4).

BODY BEAUTIFUL TECHNIQUES

Body Scrubs

Body scrubs are usually made from abrasive materials that help exfoliate dead skin cells, leaving the skin feeling soft and renewed. Body scrubs are very effective before any cellulite or slimming treatments, as body exfoliation assists with the penetration of the products. Essential oils which have cleansing properties can be used in body scrubs, such as **lemon, lemongrass, grapefruit, pine, peppermint and rosemary**.

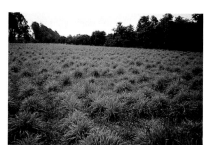

Lemongrass

Body Brushing

Body brushing (or *skin brushing*) is very popular in the East, and is used to stimulate the body and as a beauty aid. Body brushing is an excellent way to increase circulation and activate the lymphatic flow within the body. It helps with all manner of physical problems, but is particularly helpful when treating cellulite.

The brush used must be of natural, bouncy bristle, and not too harsh as this may scratch and cause discomfort. The brush strokes must be light, and in the direction of the heart. Start at the feet. Work on the back of the body, then the front.

To help eliminate cellulite, body brushing must be carried out in the direction of the lymph flow, and the entire body must be gently brushed. This method can be used before any type of slimming programme, or whenever the therapist suspects that the body's lymph flow has become sluggish.

Body brushing should be carried out on dry skin. Follow with drainage movements, using some of the body's reflex points. When that has been completed, an essential oil blend can be used in the body massage.

CELLULITE TREATMENT WITH ESSENTIAL OILS

What is Cellulite?

Normal body fat is smooth, following the outline and curves of the body. Cellulite in the adipose tissue is often found in areas that have poor circulation and elimination, such as the hips, thighs and buttocks, abdomen and in the inner part of the upper arms.

Cellulite is caused by the accumulation of waste and toxic matter becoming trapped in the tissue, leading to lack of cell nourishment, with swelling and thickening of the tissues, which often feel like scar tissue. A sluggish lymphatic system can lead to lumps and nodules of hard fat.

Even women who would not normally be considered fat, such as long-distance runners, can have areas of cellulite. It becomes more obvious with age, when the connective tissue and elastin become weakened. Cellulite is often evident in people whose weight fluctuates frequently. It can be very difficult to shift, but is not an intractable problem.

It may have taken years for the condition to have become noticeable, slowly building up over time. Cellulite is a very stubborn problem once it has taken hold, and a complete reversal of the body's functioning needs to takes place.

As well as essential oils, other methods that are useful in the treatment of cellulite are body brushing and massage, which increase circulation and lymph flow, improving the tone and texture of the skin. Regular exercise is essential. Nutrition is of the utmost importance. The client should be advised to go on a de-toxification diet, cutting out wheat and dairy products, red meats, alcohol, coffee, tea and fried foods. At the same time, they should drink plenty of water, and consider taking a vitamin and mineral supplement.

Cellulite Treatment

As removal of trapped toxins depends on a good lymphatic flow, the treatment should include a body massage.

1. *Dry skin brushing*: always follow the direction of the lymphatic flow. This can be carried out with the client either standing or sitting. The entire body should be brushed.
2. *Exfoliation*: use a natural exfoliating product, easily removable from the skin.
3. *Compress*: to help increase circulation to stubborn areas. Apply a ginger, black pepper and cardamom compress, wrapping the whole of the area to be treated.
4. *Essential oil massage*: apply essential oils diluted in vegetable carrier oil over the back, avoiding cellulite areas. Then apply the same massage oil, but at a 20 per cent higher dilution, over the stubborn cellulite areas. Massage these areas using movements that flow outwards, and incorporate the pressing of body reflex points into the massage.
    Repeat the whole process on the front of the body.
    Suitable essential oils to use in the massage oil are: **lemongrass, thyme linalol, rosemary, cypress, grapefruit, black pepper, juniper, fennel, and eucalyptus**.
5. Products can be given to the client for home use. It is advisable to suggest that skin brushing is carried out at least once a week.

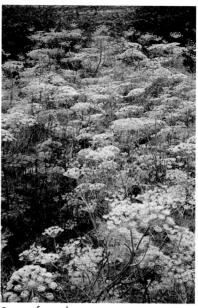
Sweet fennel

MASSAGE FOR TIRED AND ACHING LEGS

- Leg massage is effective for removing trapped cellular debris and toxins and stimulating lymphatic flow – which helps reduce oedema.
- Although massage is contra-indicated for varicose veins, a simple gentle application of diluted essential oils on the skin, using *no massage whatsoever*, is acceptable, and helpful in this condition. Use an equal combination of **cypress and geranium**.
- Tired legs benefit from massage using diluted **peppermint, rosemary and lemongrass**.

ACHING MUSCLES

Muscles ache for a variety of reasons:

- over-stimulation through work or recreational exercise;
- during illness;
- because of viral or bacterial infections that attack the nervous system and muscular structure of the body;
- because of rheumatism and other conditions.

Which essential oils are chosen for inclusion in the massage oil will depend on the cause of the aching muscles. Essential oils that could generally be used include **lavender, camomile, rosemary, thyme linalol, marjoram, black pepper and ginger**.

USING ESSENTIAL OILS IN BODY MASSAGE DURING PREGNANCY

Essential oil massage can be very beneficial during pregnancy, and regular massage can even prepare the body for an easier delivery. The woman having regular massage during pregnancy will experience fewer tense muscles, and become used to allowing the body to relax. Suitable essential oils to use at this time would be: **palmarosa, tangerine, geranium, camomile roman, rose** and **jasmine**. See page 102 for the appropriate percentage dilution to use. During labour, essential oils can be diffused in the labour or delivery rooms.

ACNE ON THE BACK AND SHOULDERS

The following treatment is intended for use on the upper back and shoulders. It should not be applied to any other area of the body.

Acne often appears on the upper back and shoulders, and in some cases the back will be almost covered in black-heads, comedones, nodules, papules, pustules, scarring/macules and white-heads.

In many clients, this area is very tense, and it is most probable that some neck releasing massage will help reduce the stress held there. However, do not massage directly over areas of acne, as this may only serve to increase any inflammation. All work carried out on this condition should be done very gently.

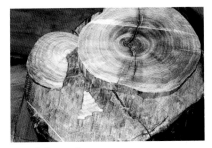

Sandalwood

1. Cleanse the back and shoulders 3–4 times. Between each cleansing, wipe with lavender hydrolat or lavender essential oil-water, applied with disposable cloths.
2. Apply the first blend of essential oils, diluted in jojoba oil. The essential oils used should have anti-bacterial and anti-inflammatory qualities. The percentage of essential oil used in this instance should be at least 5 per cent.
3. Cover the back and shoulders with a compress using a blend of lavender and camomile german hydrolats, or an essential oil water if a hydrolat is not available.
4. Apply a mask over the back and shoulders.
5. Gently smooth over the affected area your blend of diluted essential oils. Suitable oils for inclusion would be *camomile german, yarrow, geranium, rosemary, lemon, orange, thyme linalol and sandalwood.*

ESSENTIAL OILS FOR BODY TREATMENTS

Body Treatments	Relaxing	Stimulating	Revitalising	Toning	Circulation	Stress	Tension	Fatigue	Exhaustion	Depression	Insomnia	Nervous condition	Aches and pains	Stiffness	Light spasms	Cellulite	Fluid retention	Congestion	Sluggishness	Digestive problems	Eczema	Psoriasis	Acne	Skin infection	Rashes	Inflammation	Scarring	Menopause	Dysmenorrhoea	PMT
Basil		●			●			●				●	●					●												
Bergamot	●					●	●			●												●	●				●			
Black Pepper		●			●			●	●				●	●				●		●										
Bois de Rose	●		●			●	●																	●						●
Camomile German															●			●			●	●	●	●	●	●	●			
Camomile Roman	●		●			●	●				●	●	●	●									●			●				●
Cedarwood						●	●	●	●									●			●	●			●					
Clary Sage	●					●	●			●			●	●	●	●												●	●	●
Cypress		●		●	●											●	●	●										●	●	●
Eucalyptus Radiata		●		●									●	●				●	●						●	●				
Fennel	●			●												●	●			●								●	●	●
Frankincense						●	●		●	●								●						●			●			
Geranium	●		●	●	●	●	●	●		●						●	●	●									●			●
Ginger		●						●					●	●	●			●	●											
Jasmine	●		●			●	●			●																	●			
Juniper																●	●	●	●		●	●	●	●	●	●				
Lavender	●					●	●	●		●	●	●	●		●						●	●	●	●	●	●	●			●
Lemon		●				●	●	●		●						●	●						●							
Lemongrass		●			●			●							●			●	●				●							
Mandarin	●					●		●															●							
Marjoram						●	●	●					●	●	●			●												
Melissa		●				●				●		●												●	●					
Neroli	●	●				●				●	●	●															●			
Orange		●					●	●	●										●	●			●							
Palmarosa	●							●									●			●			●							
Patchouli			●		●					●						●	●	●						●	●				●	●
Peppermint		●						●	●					●	●			●	●	●						●				
Petitgrain	●					●	●		●	●	●	●			●									●						
Rose Maroc	●		●		●					●																		●	●	●
Rose Otto	●					●	●			●	●				●												●			●
Rosemary		●		●	●			●					●	●		●	●	●	●										●	
Sandalwood	●					●	●		●	●		●												●		●				
Tea Tree																							●	●	●					
Thyme Linalol		●											●	●	●			●	●				●	●						
Vetiver						●	●		●		●				●															
Violet Leaf				●			●											●					●							
Ylang-ylang	●		●	●		●	●			●		●																	●	●

CHAPTER 10

Cosmetic Surgery

Cosmetic surgery is carried out either as a necessity – a requirement of medical treatment, or as a personal choice – to enhance the look of a person. In either case, preparing the skin before surgery can in some cases be the difference between being left with unsightly scarring, or very little or even no scarring. The measures below can also be applied to other types of surgery.

A cosmetic surgeon cannot tell beforehand whether the skin of a particular individual will respond well or not to surgery, in terms of scarring. Healing is a very individual process. This can present a problem to cosmetic surgeons, who are very much concerned to provide a service that doesn't leave the patient unhappy with their looks.

Surgeons carrying out life-saving procedures are not as concerned about the look of the skin after the event, but most patients do not want to be left with a permanent reminder of the suffering they have been through. It is often the aromatherapist or beauty therapist, rather than the surgeon, who through the experience of their clients are made to realise just how distressing scarring can be to some people. Their use of essential oils in before- or after-surgery treatments may not eliminate the scar completely, but may lessen it.

PRE-OPERATIVE MEASURES

HEALTH AND SAFETY
Essential oil use is contra-indicated when the client is planning to undergo facial peeling or laser treatment, which require that certain pre-operative products prescribed by the surgeon are used.

The longer you have in which to treat the client before surgery, the better. Privately funded cosmetic surgery is usually carried out without much delay, while those having medical surgery often have a lengthy time to wait.

Treatments must be once or twice a week until surgery, and include home care. Many surgeons offer their own product ranges, and sometimes these conflict with the use of essential oils. It is vital, therefore, that if such products are being used by a client, their surgeon is advised that essential oil pre-operative treatment is planned, and permission to do so is granted, before treatment can begin. Some surgeons may prefer that no treatment is given. For these reasons, it is always wise to make yourself known to the surgeon beforehand so they are aware of the planned treatment.

Treatment

Using essential oils in treatments pre-operatively can lead to less scarring and bruising, quicker recovery time, less stress and tension and, possibly, less risk of infection. Full facial and body treatments prepare the client both physically and emotionally for the surgery. For the body, choose essential oils that have a relaxing effect. For the face, choose those that have an energising, toning effect.

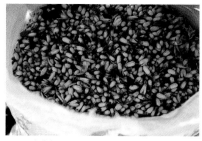

Neroli blossoms

SCARRING AND SCAR TISSUE

New Scars

- New scars respond very well to essential oil blends, which must be applied (not massaged) morning and night for full effect.
- Choose from the essential oils that are anti-inflammatory and calming, as these appear to be more effective. *Camomile, yarrow, rose and geranium* would be good choices.
- Appropriate carrier or base oils would include camellia oil, macadamia oil, evening primrose oil, red carrot oil and rosehip seed oil.

Old Scars

- Old scars take much longer to respond to treatment. Home care massage will need to be applied every day between treatments.
- Essential oils that help are *frankincense, elemi, rose, geranium, fennel, lemon, orange and carrot seed.*
- Carrier or base oils that are very useful are rosehip seed oil, borage oil, red carrot root oil and macadamia oil.
- Prepare a massage oil for the scar area using the essential oils and vegetable oils suggested above, while using a less specialised blend on the rest of the body.

HEALTH AND SAFETY
Products may be applied if the surgeon has agreed.

HEALTH AND SAFETY
Do not massage over any new scar tissue, but apply essential oils in compresses or, when suitably diluted, smooth gently over the area.

A client's general practitioner or consultant's consent should be sought before attempting any essential oil use on new scarring.

Water Treatments

Essential oils are used very successfully in water-based treatments in health spas and salons such as hydrotherapy, healing baths, saunas, steam rooms and floatation tanks. The choice of essential oil will depend on the treatment being given and the required result.

SOOTHING HEALING BATHS

Therapeutic baths can be an effective and interesting way of extending the treatments offered by a health spa or salon.

Because essential oils and water do not mix, there has been some speculation about how essential oils have a therapeutic effect in water, and some researchers believe it is by inhalation and absorption through the mucus membrane of the nose. However, essential oils also penetrate the skin by a process called osmosis, and other researchers have suggested that while in the water, the minute fatty essential oil molecules are attracted to the oily or fatty coating of the skin – following the principle of 'like attracts like'. The heat of the water opens the pores, and thus the essential oils can penetrate the epidermis.

The therapeutic value of water has been appreciated by many cultures around the world and some of these use fragrant materials in baths. In Balinese beauty treatments, for example, the client is first given a body pack made with local crushed spices, such as cardamom, ginger and turmeric, then a vigorous body massage, and finally relaxation in a bath full of beautiful, highly scented floating flowers.

If your salon has the facilities to provide fragrant warm baths, these could be given after a body massage using essential oils.

SAUNAS

In saunas using heated coals, herb or essential oil teas can be used. Add 10 ml (⅓ ounce) of a pre-prepared herbal 'tea' or essential oil 'water' (see Chapter Four, page 33) in the bucket holding the water that is thrown over the coals. They will impart a gentle, cleansing fragrance to the atmosphere. The traditional essential oils to use are *pine, fir, eucalyptus or rosemary*. To create a fresh, clean, and less medicinal aroma, add an additional 10 drops of *grapefruit, lemon or orange* to each litre of water when making the 'water'.

STEAM ROOMS

If intending to use essential oil in the water container in the machinery used in steam rooms, consult the manufacturer to ensure that essential oils are compatible. However, simply leaving a hot herbal 'tea' in a bowl in the room will help to create a pleasing fragrance; or use *grapefruit, lemon, orange, pine, fir, eucalyptus or rosemary* essential oil 'waters'.

HOSING DOWN AND UNDER-WATER MASSAGE

If using the water hosing down method, under-water jet air pressure or under-water manual massage, essential oils can be used before treatment – diluted in a vegetable carrier oil and applied to the body. Use essential oils appropriate for the purpose of the water treatment being given, choosing from the essential oil profiles.

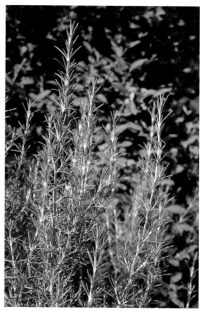

Rosemary

CHAPTER 12

Essential Oils and Hair Removal

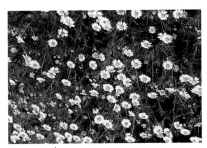

Camomile german

Essential oils are used in hair removal treatments mainly for their calming, soothing, anti-bacterial and anti-fungal effects on the skin. They can also be useful applied in a lotion as an anti-inflammatory agent to help prevent redness, and to close the pores – after waxing for example.

EPILATION

After traditional epilation techniques, a gel is usually applied. These sometimes contain witch hazel, which is used to calm down the skin and, being slightly astringent, helps close the pores. Certain essential oils can also perform these functions and can be mixed into any sterile gel which is used for after-care. *Tea tree, manuka, lavender and lemon* essential oils are antiseptic, and will help reduce the risk of cross-infection.

WAXING

Many waxing products now being used include essential oils and vegetable oils to reduce skin problems during waxing, and help the skin recover after the hairs have been removed. After-care lotions often contain essential oils to help reduce redness and other waxing problems, however they will not be able to help any allergic reaction to the wax.

Essential oils that would be helpful when included in sterile or purpose-made lotions and gels after waxing treatments are those such as *camomile german, camomile roman, lavender, tea tree, manuka and palmarosa.*

Sensitive skin appears to respond to waxing by becoming more sensitive for a while, and in some women a *camomile german and lavender combination* can help to calm the redness.

HEALTH AND SAFETY
Essential oils in hair-removal after-care is contra-indicated for those women who are sensitive or allergic to highly perfumed products and essential oils, while special care must be taken with women who have highly sensitive skins (see right).

SUGARING

In times past, sugaring was carried out using sugar and lemon juice and in some Middle Eastern countries today, beauty therapists still use this method but add the essential oil of lemon too. In after-care products, the essential oils of **lemon and rosemary** can be used. As some Middle Eastern women must remove all body hair, care must be taken in these cases to ensure that no essential oil falls on delicate genital mucus membrane.

THREADING

In tea or floral-water form, essential oils can be used both before and after threading, as they are said to assist in the thread gripping on the hair, and reduce redness afterwards. Appropriate suggestions before threading would be the citrus essential oils such as **lemon, lime and grapefruit**. As after-care, use **lavender and camomile german**.

CHAPTER 13

Hands, Feet and Nails

The hands and feet benefit from treatments containing essential oils, as much as any other part of the body does. As well as beautifying and providing protection, they can help in the healing of wounds and burns, and effectively deal with viral or fungal infection.

Certain vegetable oils are often the only ingredient in some of the most exclusive and expensive fingernail treatments for softening cuticles, rectifying splitting or flaking nails, strengthening them and encouraging new growth.

Together, essential oils and vegetable oils provide the tools for effective hand treatments. They are used in hand massage, intensive hand therapy, as well as in treatments for specific conditions such as eczema, psoriasis, warts, infections, wounds and burns.

HAND MASSAGE CREAMS

The hand creams and lotions used on clients in the salon environment should be able to fulfil specific requirements. But often they are no different from the general products commercially available on the retail market. However, by using appropriate essential oils and vegetable oils, the therapist or nail technician has the tools to perform the following tasks:

- *soften the skin*
- *tone the skin*
- *help reduce the visible signs of ageing*
- *heal broken skin*
- *reduce any fluid congestion in the hands and fingers*
- *soothe aching muscles*

Basic Hand Cream Recipe

The following ingredients can be blended to make a basic hand cream. Add to it 10 drops of essential oil, choosing from the essential oil profiles on pages 39–75, depending on the function you wish the cream to perform.

15 g (½ oz) cocoa butter
40 ml (1⅓ oz) almond oil
15 g (½ oz) beeswax
5 drops of evening primrose oil
5 drops of carrot oil

Melt the cocoa butter and the beeswax in a bain-marie/double-boiler, then add the almond, evening primrose and carrot oils. Mix together well. This basic hand cream can be made thinner by adding more almond oil, or thicker by including less almond oil at the outset. Add 10 drops of essential oil when the blend is complete, and mix in well.

The following essential oils can be added to the basic hand cream above, or to vegetable oils, or to products especially designed for the addition of essential oils. Your choice of essential oils will depend on the specific function you require of the hand massage product, and is not limited to those below:

geranium, lemon, rose, palmarosa, peppermint and lavender.

WARTS

Warts on the fingers and hands are very common and are often difficult to eradicate. As warts are caused by a virus, anti-viral essential oils are used in their treatment. Refer to *The Fragrant Pharmacy* (for details see *Further Reading* in the Appendix at the end of this book).

NAILS

Full-time aromatherapists have no trouble with their own nails, which grow strong and long because of the constant contact with essential oils. Indeed, aromatherapy students often lament the irony of the fact that even though their nails have become beautifully healthy, they have to be kept trimmed so that treatments can be performed. Fixed vegetable oils also play an important role in nail care, those listed on the right are particularly effective.

These suggestions will be helpful in cases when the nails are discoloured and appear unhealthy, which is often because the nails have been continuously covered with varnish for long periods of time, or following acrylic nail removal.

When nails become soft and unhealthy they are at risk of infections, including fungal infection. Suggested essential oils in this instance would be:

manuka, tea tree, lavender, lemon, thyme linalol and lemongrass.

NAIL PRODUCTS – HEALTH AND SAFETY ISSUES

There is a very strong case for using natural products wherever possible in nail care. Nail technicians may be aware that there is much debate, especially in the USA, regarding the safety of synthetic chemicals used in commercially available nail care products. This is of particular concern to those working with acrylic and other false nails. Although the subject of health and safety is largely directed at client care, it is the therapist working with these chemicals on a daily basis who is at greater risk.

> **NAILBED TREATMENT VEGETABLE OILS**
> jojoba, rosehip seed, borage, apricot kernel

> **CUTICLE SOFTENING VEGETABLE OILS**
> avocado, wheatgerm, red carrot root

If a client or therapist experiences problems with their health, or has an adverse skin or nail reaction to treatment, it is possible that this is being caused by the chemicals in the products. At the centre of the debate is methyl methacrylate (MMA), which has been accused of causing the following problems: allergies and MMA intolerance, toxicity, loss of nail, damaged nailbed, dry, flaking or splitting nails. Problems have also been reported regarding the fingers themselves, although this is rare.

If working with false nails on a regular basis, the therapist or nail technician should be aware of the potential problems attributed to the following chemicals often found in nail related products:

methyl methacrylate (MMA)	headaches; dizziness; toxicity; dry hands; itching; rashes; allergies; MMA intolerance
acetone	skin irritation; rashes; dry patches on hands or other areas of body, if touched
benzoyl peroxide	used in anti-infection products to treat nail and hand infections: can be very harsh on sensitive and delicate skin; inflammation
formaldehyde	toxic if fumes are inhaled; headaches; dizziness; faintness; nausea
hydroquinone	used in anti-ageing creams and brown-spot treatment creams: rashes; redness; dry skin
oleic acid	skin rashes; itching

THE FEET

When essential oils are used in foot treatments, they help stimulate the circulation and refresh, or relax, the whole body. Treatment can begin with a foot bath, using a cleansing product that contains essential oils with anti-bacterial and anti-fungal action. If this is not available, simply add essential oils with those properties to the water, or in hydrolat or essential oil 'water' form.

As so many foot infections are picked up by walking barefoot in public areas, such as swimming pools, gyms and even beauty salons, anti-bacterial and anti-fungal essential oils can be used in foot treatments, whether the client has a problem or not.

If intending to use any essential oil products in conjunction with electrical foot-bath equipment, first check with the manufacturer.

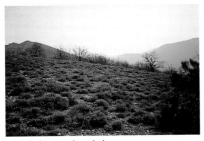
Wild thyme linalol

Hydrolats

Following a foot bath, dry the feet and spray with a refreshing hydrolat. This prepares the feet for the next step of the pedicure.

Foot Massage

Essential oils can be diluted in fixed vegetable oils, or added to creams or lotions designed for use with essential oils, including:

tea tree, manuka, thyme linalol, nutmeg, grapefruit, rosemary, spearmint and frankincense.

Cuticles and Hard Skin Removal

Fixed vegetable oils, with or without essential oils, can be used to soften cuticles, or after the removal of hard skin.

Nailbed Infections

Apply neat *tea tree or manuka* on the end of a cotton bud.

Verrucas and Athlete's Foot

It is not within the scope of beauty therapy to treat these conditions, however essential oils can be very effective in these areas. Refer the client to *The Fragrant Pharmacy* (for details see *Further Reading* in the Appendix at the end of this book).

FOOT MASSAGE

The feet are extremely well supplied with nerve endings. Reflexology utilises this fact to stimulate precise areas of the foot that correspond to organs and certain areas of the muscular and skeletal system. Aromatherapy treatments often include reflexology.

When a therapist massages the feet, they are working in an area that is so complex that it constitutes of itself an entire branch of complementary medicine – reflexology – which requires specialist training. However, all clients can benefit from gentle foot massage that does not involve movements that press too deeply into the tissue. Use essential oils that have an effect on the whole body, by being either relaxing or stimulating, as the client requests.

The Working Environment – Health and Safety in the Salon

RELEVANT BRITISH LAWS

The following Acts may be relevant to using essential oils in your workplace. Enquire at your local library, where copies of the applicable documents may be held.

Health and Safety at Work Act 1974
Health and Safety (First Aid) Regulations 1981
The Management of Health and Safety at Work Regulations 1992
Control of Substances Hazardous to Health Act 1994
Fire Precautions Act 1971
Office, Shop and Railway Premises Act 1963
Electricity at Work Regulations 1990
Local Government (Miscellaneous Provisions) Act 1982
The Industry Code of Practice for Hygiene in Beauty Salons and Clinics
Consumer Protection Act 1987
Sale of Goods and Services Act 1982
Trades Description Act 1968 and 1972

The salon or independent therapist may require:

Employer's liability insurance (1969 Act)
Public liability insurance
Product liability insurance
Professional indemnity insurance

The Medicines Act 1968

The Medicines Act states that no medicinal claim can be made for an essential oil or essential oil product (on the label, in advertisements or promotional literature), unless a special licence has been obtained. It costs millions of pounds to provide the licensing authorities with the required medical trials to back up any such claim. Consequently, few licences are applied for by the aromatherapy trade.

Spots are considered a medical condition under the law, along with minor conditions such as colds, cuts and bruises, as well as the more serious conditions, such as rheumatism. It is illegal, in the absence of a licence, for a supplier to provide you with an essential oil or essential oil product that claims to be able to cure spots, or cure any other condition, illness or disease. Likewise, it is illegal for you to make such claims for products supplied by yourself or the salon.

If you produce an aromatherapy product for sale, you must refer to *A Guide to the Cosmetic Products (Safety) Regulations* (see below). Although the product label or literature cannot claim to cure anything, it can state that the product can:

- clean;
- perfume;
- change the appearance;
- protect;
- keep in good condition;
- correct body odour.

In addition, it can be stated that

- '[name of product] can be used for/on…'.

A Guide to the Cosmetic Products (Safety) Regulations

This booklet is available from the Consumer Safety Unit at your local Department of Trade and Industry office, or from the main office in London (see Appendix at the end of this book for details). It is the essential guide when producing products for sale. Within the European Community, laws in this area are often changing, and it is wise to keep up to date.

Knowledge Review

INTRODUCTION – AESTHETIC AROMATHERAPY

1. What is the distinction between aesthetic aromatherapy and clinical aromatherapy?
2. Fragrance has been used by many cultures throughout history. Name three such cultures, and describe the ways in which they used fragrance.
3. Name two methods used by ancient cultures to extract essential oils from plant materials.
4. Who coined the term 'aromatherapy'?
5. Who introduced the use of essential oils and aromatherapy as a beauty treatment?
6. Essential oils are used in several distinct therapies or purposes. Name four, and describe how they are used in each.
7. From the *Glossary of Therapeutic Properties*, choose 15 examples that are useful in beauty therapy. Give the name of the therapeutic property in medical terminology, followed by a brief explanation of its physical effect.

CHAPTER 1 – HOW AROMATHERAPY WORKS

1. Name five physiological effects of aromatherapy.
2. Name two psychological effects of aromatherapy.
3. In beauty therapy, essential oils work on the body and mind in two ways. Name them.
4. Describe the mechanism of olfaction.
5. The olfactory system is part of which organ?
6. What term describes the permanent loss of the sense of smell?
7. Name six functions performed by the skin.
8. Explain the structure of skin.
9. Essential oils are thought to travel through the body. How is that at present thought to happen?
10. How do essential oils affect the following systems? Also name two essential oils that are thought to have an effect on each.
    (a) Circulatory/cardiovascular system
    (b) Lymphatic system
    (c) Nervous system
    (d) Endocrine system
    (e) Muscular system

(f) Digestive system
(g) Respiratory system
(h) Reproductive system
(i) Skeletal system.

CHAPTER 2 – SAFETY AND CONTRA-INDICATIONS

1. Name four steps that a therapist should take to ensure their safety while working with essential oils.
2. What do you do if essential oils get into the eyes?
3. What do you do if skin irritation occurs after applying diluted essential oils?
4. What safety measure should you take when blending essential oils?
5. (a) What is the term given to a local reaction of the skin to certain substances?
   (b) Name four essential oils which are known to cause this reaction, and should not be applied to the skin.
   (c) Name ten essential oils which should be used with care on sensitive skins.
6. (a) What is the term given to an allergic reaction to certain substances?
   (b) Name two essential oils that should be avoided by people with allergic reactions.
7. (a) What is the term given to the photo-chemical reaction of the skin caused by direct ultra-violet (UV) rays of the sun?
   (b) Which is the main group of essential oils that cause this reaction?
   (c) Name four essential oils from this group.
   (d) Name three other essential oils not from this group that should not be applied to the skin before exposure to UV light.
8. Name ten essential oils that should not be used under any circumstances.
9. Name ten essential oils that should be avoided by women who are pregnant or breast-feeding.
10. Name six essential oils that should not be used on those who are prone to epilepsy.
11. How do you extinguish fire involving essential oils?

CHAPTER 3 – FIXED VEGETABLE OILS

1. Vegetable oils are obtained from two sources.
   (a) Name them
   (b) Give two examples of each.
2. Give two physical characteristics of fixed vegetable oils.
3. Explain the difference between a 'carrier' oil and a 'base' oil.
4. The best quality vegetable oils are produced in certain ways. Give four examples of those processes.
5. Name two disadvantages of using highly processed vegetable oils.

6. Certain fixed vegetable oils are more suitable for specific skin types. Which skin types are the following five oils particularly suitable for:

   (a) Almond
   (b) Avocado
   (c) Grapeseed
   (d) Hazelnut
   (e) Jojoba.

CHAPTER 4 – ESSENTIAL OILS AND HYDROLATS

1. Name three reasons why a plant might produce essential oils.
2. Essential oils are stored in different parts of plants, depending on the species. Name ten such places.
3. Name three physical characteristics of essential oils.
4. What causes essential oils to change consistency?
5. Essential oils vary in colour. Name two oils which are:
   (a) colourless
   (b) yellow-orange
   (c) blue.
6. Name two oils that are:
   (a) fluid
   (b) viscous.
7. Perfumers describe fragrances as having a certain 'note'. Name the three types of note.
8. For what reasons are essential oils placed in each fragrance 'note' category?
9. Name four methods by which essential oils are extracted from plant materials.
10. Describe the process of steam distillation.
11. How are hydrolats produced?
12. Name one hydrolat that can be used for:
    (a) softening
    (b) refreshing
    (c) stimulating
    (d) balancing
    (e) soothing
    (f) acne/spots
    (g) inflammation.
13. Explain the difference between hydrolats and essential oil 'waters'.
14. Essential oils consist of various groups of chemicals. Name five such chemical groups.
15. Name four ways in which essential oils might be adulterated, giving a brief description of each.
16. Name three ways in which the purity of essential oils can be ensured.
17. Name two methods by which the chemical constituents of essential oils are tested for.

The Essential Oil Beauty Profiles

18. Name four essential oils listed in the profiles that should not be used in facial treatments.

19. Name one essential oil that can be used in facial treatments for:
    (a) acne
    (b) ageing skin
    (c) blemishes
    (d) broken capillaries
    (e) combination skin
    (f) congestion
    (g) dry skin
    (h) inflamed skin
    (i) mature skin
    (j) normal skin
    (k) oily skin
    (l) open pores
    (m) revitalisation
    (n) scarring
    (o) sensitive skin
    (p) skin tone
    (q) sluggishness.

20. Name one essential oil that can be used in body treatments for:
    (a) balancing
    (b) cellulite
    (c) circulation
    (d) congestion
    (e) diuretic
    (f) fatigue
    (g) general aches
    (h) muscle tone
    (i) relaxation
    (j) revitalisation
    (k) sluggishness
    (l) stiffness
    (m) stimulation
    (n) stress
    (o) tension
    (p) tonic.

21. Name the contra-indications of the following essential oils:
    (a) basil
    (b) bergamot
    (c) black pepper
    (d) clary sage
    (e) fennel
    (f) ginger
    (g) juniper berry
    (h) lemon
    (i) peppermint
    (j) rosemary
    (k) thyme linalol.

CHAPTER 5 – PROFESSIONAL BLENDING TECHNIQUES

1. When blending the ingredients for a base or carrier oil, do you start with the smallest or largest amount?
2. When blending essential oils, do you start with the smallest or largest amount?
3. Name at least six pieces of equipment used in the making of aromatherapy blends.
4. Give two reasons why is it important to have blending sheets for pre-prepared blends.
5. To create a pleasant fragrance, what are the fragrance 'notes' that require consideration when making an essential oil blend?
6. Name at least ten items of information that should be listed on a client's blend sheet.
7. Name at least six points to consider when choosing essential oils to use on a particular client.
8. What must you do after giving a client a blend to use at home?
9. What type of insurance is required to be able to blend essential oils for clients?

CHAPTER 6 – THE SALON AND RETAIL SALES POTENTIAL

1. Name four ways in which essential oils can be used in the salon environment.
2. How long does an essential oil retain its therapeutic value, on average?
3. Why is it important to ventilate the treatment room between each client?
4. Give three reasons why essential oils should not be used in a diffuser in the treatment room.
5. What two steps can the therapist take to prevent an accumulation of essential oils in her body?
6. When carrying out aromatherapy facial or body treatments with pre-prepared products, name three additional pieces of equipment that should be available in the treatment room.
7. If carrying out individualised aromatherapy facial or body treatments, what equipment, additional to the three in 6. above, should be available?
8. Why is it important to wash hands between each stage of the treatment?
9. Name eight essential oils which have no toxicological possibilities, and are safe to use during pregnancy, on children and for general home care, and are therefore suitable for retail sale.
10. What are the four key points to remember about essential oil storage?

CHAPTER 7 – CLIENT CARE

1. In the case of facial treatment, what four steps constitute the client assessment?

2. What six broad areas should the consultation cover?
3. Give ten examples of things you would look for when making a facial skin examination.
4. Name ten skin conditions that may have resulted from the use of medications.

CHAPTER 8 – AROMATHERAPY FOR FACIAL TREATMENTS

1. Name nine ways in which essential oils can be used in facial treatments.
2. When treating the face, are any other parts of the body affected, and why?
3. Give three reasons why the psychological benefits of essential oils can be more fully realised during a facial in the salon environment.
4. What dilution of essential oils would be used in the following cases? Give the minimum and maximum amounts.
   (a) Sensitive skin
   (b) Acne
   (c) Emotional state
   (d) On medication (generally)
   (e) Pregnancy.
5. How do you make and use a herbal or floral tea compress?
6. Give one example of an appropriate herbal compress for the following skin types:
   (a) dry
   (b) sensitive
   (c) normal
   (d) mature
   (e) acne.
7. List the five benefits of a facial massage incorporating essential oils.
8. Name four techniques that are used in a basic essential oil facial massage.
9. What has a relaxing effect in aesthetic aromatherapy?
10. What assists the energy-flow to the client?
11. When would facial massage be contra-indicated?
12. What eight steps does an aromatherapy facial consist of?
13. Why is cleansing particularly important in aromatherapy facials?
14. Why are facial tonics used?
15. Why are herbal compresses or poultices used?
16. Which essential oils can be used after the extraction of blackheads?
17. Which essential oils can be used on spots or blemishes?
18. Which products should be avoided if the client has a wheat or nut allergy?
19. List the nine acne treatment steps.
20. How many acne treatments should a client have during:
    (a) weeks 1–2
    (b) weeks 3–4
    (c) weeks 6–13?

21. What home-care should be suggested after acne treatment facials?

22. Which essential oils would be appropriate choices for use in facials, with the following skin types?
(a) Normal
(b) Dry
(c) Oily
(d) Sensitive
(e) Mature.

CHAPTER 9 – ESSENTIAL OIL BODY TREATMENTS

1. Name five purposes for which body massage treatments might be carried out.

2. Put the word 'body' or 'face' into the spaces:
All essential oils that are used on the ...., can be used on the .... but not all essential oils used on the .... can be used on the ....

3. Generally, what percentage of essential oil should be used in a diluted blend for the following? Give the minimum and maximum amounts.
(a) For general relaxation
(b) Body massage
(c) When treating a specific condition, or aches or pains, during slimming, cellulite or toning treatments.

4. Give three examples when less than the amounts in 3. above would be used?

5. When carrying out a skin analysis of the body, what may be indicated by the following:
(a) pale skin
(b) discoloured areas
(c) yellowish skin or with poor pallor
(d) bluish tinge
(e) cold hands and feet
(f) varicose veins
(g) spongy tissue
(h) tension in the muscles
(i) knotted fibrous tissue
(j) hard and congested areas
(k) thickened toe nails.

6. Name six essential oils that would be suitable choices in a massage for cellulite treatment.

7. Name six essential oils that would be suitable to use in a body massage during pregnancy.

8. Name three essential oils that could be used on aching muscles.

9. List two essential oils that are appropriate choices in aromatherapy massage for:
(a) relaxation
(b) stress
(c) tension
(d) toning
(e) stimulation.

CHAPTER 10 – COSMETIC SURGERY

1. Why are essential oils contra-indicated when a client is planning to undergo facial peeling or laser treatment?
2. When is it contra-indicated to massage over scar tissue?
3. What replacement treatment can be used if massage is contra-indicated?
4. Which essential oils assist in improving the appearance of old scarring?
5. Which base oils assist in improving the appearance of old scarring?

CHAPTER 11 – WATER TREATMENTS

1. Which essential oils are contra-indicated in water methods, and why?
2. Name three mediums in which essential oils can be diluted for use in water treatment methods.
3. It has been suggested that essential oils penetrate the skin while in water by a process called 'osmosis'. Explain this process.

CHAPTER 12 – ESSENTIAL OILS AND HAIR REMOVAL

1. Give four reasons why essential oils can be beneficial in hair removal treatments.
2. Name four essential oils that are suitable for incorporation in epilation after-care gels.
3. Name six essential oils that are suitable for incorporation in after-waxing lotions and gels.
4. Name two essential oils that can be used in 'tea' or 'floral water' form:
   (a) before threading
   (b) after threading.

CHAPTER 13 – HANDS, FEET AND NAILS

1. Name six effects that can be achieved by using appropriate vegetable oils and essential oils in hand treatments.
2. List three vegetable oils suitable for nailbed treatment.
3. List three vegetable oils suitable for cuticle softening.
4. List three essential oils that can assist in the healing of fungal infections of the nails.
5. List three essential oils that are appropriate for use in foot baths.
6. List three essential oils that are appropriate for use in foot massage.
7. Which complementary medicine is carried out on the feet?

FURTHER READING

Battaglia, Salvatore, *The Complete Guide to Aromatherapy* (Virginia, The Perfect Potion Pty Ltd, 1995)

Duke, James A., *The Green Pharmacy* (Rodale Press, 1997)

Gattefossé, René-Maurice, *Gattefossé's Aromatherapy* (Saffron Walden, Essex: C. W. Daniel Co. Ltd, 1993)

Lawless, Julia, *The Encyclopaedia of Essential Oils* (Shaftsbury, Element Books, 1997)

Lis-Balchin, Dr Maria, *Aroma Science, The Chemistry and Bioactivity of Essential Oils* (East Horsley, Amberwood, 1995)

Maury, Marguerite, *Guide to Aromatherapy – the Secret of Life and Youth* (Saffron Walden, Essex: C. W. Daniel Co. Ltd, 1989)

Valnet, Dr Jean, *The Practice of Aromatherapy* (Saffron Walden, Essex: C. W. Daniel Co. Ltd, 1980)

Worwood, Valerie Ann, *The Fragrant Pharmacy* (London, Bantam Books, 1991)

Worwood, Valerie Ann, *The Fragrant Mind* (London, Bantam Books, 1997)

Worwood, Valerie Ann, *The Fragrant Heavens* (London, Bantam Books, 1999)

Worwood, Valerie Ann, *Aromatherapy for the Healthy Child* (Novato USA, New World Library, 1999)

Williams, David G., *The Chemistry of Essential Oils* (Weymouth, Micelle Press, 1996)

ORGANISATIONS

The International Federation of Aromatherapists (IFA)
Stamford House
182 Chiswick High Road
London W4
Telephone: 0208-742 2605
www.int-fed-aromatherapy.co.uk
Examines aromatherapists; membership includes insurance. Represents professional aromatherapists.

Register of Qualified Aromatherapists
PO Box 6941
London W8 9HF
Represents professional aromatherapists; membership includes
insurance.

The International Society of Professional Aromatherapists (ISPA)
ISPA House
82 Ashby Road
Hinckley
Leics.
LE10 1SN
Telephone: 01455 637987
Represents professional aromatherapists; membership includes
insurance.

Hairdressing and Beauty Industry Authority (HABIA)
The National Training Organisation for Hairdressing and Beauty
Therapy
2nd Floor, Fraser House
Nether Hall Road
Doncaster DN1 2PH
Telephone: 01302 380000
www.habia.org.uk

The Stationery Office (TSO)
The Publications Centre
PO Box 276
London SW8 5DT
Telephone: 08706 005522
Fax: 0870 6005533
www.tsonline.co.uk
Sells copies of all government laws, guidelines and reports.

ESSENTIAL OIL SUPPLIERS

Earth Garden
2 Fairview Parade
Mawney Road
Romford
Essex RM7 7HH
Telephone: 01708 722633

lavendin **10**, **11**
lecithin 25
leg massage 132
legal regulations 92–3, **93**, 145–6
lemon *2, 56*
   acne (back/shoulders) 133
   body treatments 130, 134
   epilation 139
   essential oil profile 56
   extraction (expression) 31
   facial treatments 120
   hair treatment xx
   hand massage cream 142
   home use 89
   life span 92
   lymphatic system 5
   nail treatments 142
   photosensitivity 11
   plant part used 27
   saunas 138
   scars 136
   starter kit **29**
   steam rooms 138
   sugaring 139–40
   threading 140
   water treatments **137**
lemongrass *57, 130*
   acne (face) 117
   body treatments 130, 134
   cellulite 132
   essential oil profile 57
   facial treatments 117, 120
   leg treatments 132
   nail treatments 142
   plant part used 27
   skin irritation 10
   substitution (adulteration) 36
life span of essential oils 92
lifestyle form 96
lime 11, 31, 92, **137**, 140
limeflowers 105
linden blossom 32
linoleic acid 25
Local Government (Miscellaneous
   Provisions) Act 1982 145
lymphatic system 5, *5*

macadamia nut oil
   base oil profile 20
   scars (new) 136
   scars (old) 136
   starter kit 102, **102**
mace **11**
macerated vegetable oils 24–5
maceration (essential oils) 30–1
Management of Health and Safety at
   Work Regulations 1992 145
mandarin *58*
   body treatments 134
   colour 28
   essential oil profile 58
   extraction (expression) 3

facial treatments 120
   home use 89
   life span 92
   photosensitivity 11
   plant part used 27
manuka *28*
   epilation 139
   foot massage 144
   nail treatments 142
   nailbed infections 144
   waxing 139
marigold *see* calendula
marjoram *59*
   body treatments 134
   essential oil profile 59
   muscle treatments 6, 132
   plant part used 26
   pregnancy/lactation **11**
marketing of essential oils/oil
   products 93, 145–6
marshmallow 105
massage
   see also body massage; facial
     massage
   energy transference 129, *129*
   foot 143–4
   scar tissue **136**
   under-water 138
massage products 122, 141–2
Maury, Marguerite xix–xx
measuring equipment **77**
medical conditions
   contra-indications **10**, 102, **129**
   marketing/advertising 146
   treatment of 9, **84**, 115
medications
   dilution of oils 102
   facial treatments **112**
   skin side-effects 97–8, 102, 116–17
Medicines Act 1968 145–6
melaleuca species 36
melissa *60*
   body treatments 134
   colour 28
   compresses 105
   essential oil profile 60
   facial treatments 120
   hydrolat 32
   substitution (adulteration) 36
methyl methacrylate (MMA) 143
mixing essential oils
   adulteration 36
   blending 76–85, 130
MMA (methyl methacrylate) 143
modern aromatherapy xviii–xix
modesty, client 125–6
moisturisers 115
mugwort **11**
muscles: aching 132
muscular system 6
mustard **11**

myrrh
   colour 28
   plant part used 27
   pregnancy/lactation **11**
   religious services xvi
   and temperature 29
   viscosity 29
myrtle 7, 27, 32, 117

nail products 142–3
nails 141, 142, **142**, 144
natural vegetable oils 13, **99**
nature-identicals 35
neroli (orange blossom) *27, 28, 29,*
   61, 136
   body treatments 134
   compresses 105
   essential oil profile 61
   facial treatments 120
   fragrance 27
   hydrolat 32
   plant part used 26, 27
   starter kit **29**
   substitution (adulteration) 36
   viscosity 29
nerve connections 127–9
nervous system 5
neutralisation of vegetable oils 14
niaouli 5, **11**
notes (aroma evaporation) 28
nut allergies 102, 115
nutmeg **11**, 144

oat 105
Office, Shop and Railway Premises Act
   1963 145
oleic acid 143
olfactory system 2, *2*
oral ingestion of essential oils 11
orange *27, 62*
   acne (back/shoulders) 133
   body treatments 134
   essential oil profile 62
   facial treatments 120
   life span 92
   photosensitivity 11
   plant part used 27
   saunas 138
   scars 136
   steam rooms 138
orange blossom *see* neroli
orange tree 27, *27*
oregano 10, **11**
organic oils 13, **37**
organisations 155–6
out-of-date essential oils **86**
ownership of blends **79**

palmarosa *63*
   body treatments **132**, 134
   essential oil profile 63
   facial treatments 120
   hand massage cream 142

GUILDFORD **college**

Learning Resource Centre

Please return on or before the last date shown.
No further issues or renewals if any items are overdue.

1 8 OCT 2006

1 3 APR 2015

Class: 615·321 WOR

Title: Aromatherapy for the...

Author: Warwood, Valerie Ann